# Basic Audiometry Learning Manual

## Second Edition

**Editor-in-Chief for Audiology**
Brad A. Stach, PhD

# Basic Audiometry Learning Manual

## *Second Edition*

**Mark DeRuiter, MBA, PhD**
**Virginia Ramachandran, AuD, PhD**

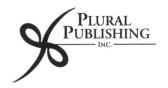

PLURAL
PUBLISHING
INC.

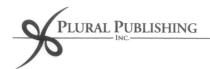

PLURAL PUBLISHING
INC.

5521 Ruffin Road
San Diego, CA 92123

e-mail: info@pluralpublishing.com
Website: http://www.pluralpublishing.com

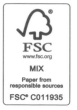

FSC
www.fsc.org
MIX
Paper from
responsible sources
FSC® C011935

Names: DeRuiter, Mark, author. | Ramachandran, Virginia, author.
Title: Basic audiometry learning manual / Mark DeRuiter, Virginia
  Ramachandran.
Other titles: Core clinical concepts in audiology.
Description: Second edition. | San Diego, CA : Plural Publishing, [2017] |
  Series: Core clinical concepts in audiology | Includes bibliographical
  references and index.
Identifiers: LCCN 2015037114 | ISBN 9781597568654 (alk. paper) | ISBN
  1597568651 (alk. paper)
Subjects: | MESH: Audiometry—methods.
Classification: LCC RF294 | NLM WV 272 | DDC 617.8/075—dc23
LC record available at http://lccn.loc.gov/2015037114

# Contents

# Preface

The *Basic Audiometry Learning Manual*, a volume in the Core Clinical Concepts in Audiology Series, is designed to provide beginning clinicians and students with experiences and instruction in the art and science of clinical audiometry techniques. Learning outcomes, review of concepts, observation exercises, guided practice, and review materials serve as catalysts for active learning of concepts and provide opportunity for utilization of fundamental audiometry methods.

The *Learning Manual* can be used in conjunction with a text of the instructor's choosing, or with the books of the complementary Core Clinical Concepts in Audiology: Basic Audiometry Series to promote reflection, application, and assessment of learned information. The comprehensive content of the *Learning Manual* encompasses the breadth of audiologic evaluation, including history taking and patient communication, ear canal assessment, immittance, pure-tone testing, masking, speech audiometry, otoacoustic emissions, and patient counseling. Along with its family of texts in the Core Clinical Concepts in Audiology Series, the *Learning Manual* is designed to cultivate successful learning by students and professionals.

Each chapter of the *Learning Manual* consists of various components designed to guide the reader through an engaging process of active learning. The first component, Learning Outcomes, provides the reader with clear goals for knowledge and skill building and a foundation for readers to evaluate their progress toward clinical competence outcomes.

The second component, Review of Concepts, provides a concise review of the theoretical knowledge necessary for performance of clinical activities. This section provides examples that serve as a preparation for practice of the clinical skill.

The third component, Observation, challenges readers to witness the behavior of seasoned professionals in the act of clinical practice. Observation exercises may be performed by watching clinical instructors or practicing professionals in the laboratory, classroom, or clinic, utilizing the pertinent techniques with patients, students, or volunteers. The Observation component encourages students to learn by example and provides the opportunity for instructors to model exemplary clinical behavior.

The fourth component, Guided Practice, leads the reader step-by-step through exercises designed to provide first-hand experience performing clinical activities. Components of each clinical activity are segmented into manageable modules, allowing readers to experience success with the individual elements of clinical techniques and systematically guide readers toward clinical competence.

The final component, Reflection and Review, provides readers with opportunities to incorporate newfound understanding gained through Observation and Guided Practice into their theoretical and conceptual knowledge base through answering reflective and review questions. By explaining methods, describing experiences, and answering questions related to techniques, readers will demonstrate their understanding of concepts and have opportunity to assess learning in relation to expected outcomes, set forth in the Learning Outcomes section.

Chapters of the *Learning Manual* can be completed in a serial fashion, following the sequence of a typical audiologic evaluation. Alternatively, the order of activities can be tailored to suit a particular instructional curriculum, or as individual topics coalesce with the reader's immediate goals. Topics addressed in each chapter are explored in-depth in the books of the associated Basic Audiometry Series of the Core Clinical Concepts in Audiology Series, and references are provided to these books to provide an integrated learning experience for readers. Readers may also find additional information from other sources as well to be used as a supplement to or in lieu of these texts.

We wish to thank all the individuals who have assisted in the process of the creation of this book. We sincerely appreciate the opportunity to create this *Learning Manual* as a component of the series. We appreciate the efforts of all of the individuals at Plural Publishing who have guided us through the publishing process. We also thank those users of the first edition who provided valuable feedback regarding suggested modifications for the second edition of this text.

It is our sincere hope that instructors and students will find the material in this book helpful in their quest for translating theoretical material into clinical skills.

*We gratefully dedicate this book to our families who have supported us through and through:*

Cathy DeRuiter and Matthew DeRuiter
Karthik Ramachandran and Nathan Ramachandran

# ‖ 1 ‖

## Greeting the Patient

In this chapter, you will learn how to greet patients and set expectations for the evaluation process in a professional manner. Once you have learned the fundamentals of greeting a patient and explaining the evaluation process, you will be able to build on this knowledge to develop your own style in interacting with patients and their families.

## LEARNING OUTCOMES

■ Be able to greet patients appropriately.
■ Be able to explain what will happen during the evaluation process.

## REVIEW OF CONCEPTS

### Greeting the Patient

Many factors come into play when greeting a patient for the first time. For the most part, patients will see you before they speak to you. Therefore,

your physical appearance is crucial. Do you look the part of the professional in the environment? Are you suitably dressed and wearing appropriate identification to reveal your role? Overall, your appearance should set you apart as belonging in the health care environment.

Observe whether anyone is accompanying the patient. Many patients who have difficulty hearing will bring a companion to assist with communication. Ask the patient if he or she would like this person to be present with them during the examination. If the accompanying person is an interpreter, remember some important factors:

■ While the interpretation is occurring, speak to the patient rather than the interpreter.
■ Verify whether the interpreter will be interpreting sequentially (after you speak) or simultaneously (while you are speaking). If the interpreter will be using a sequential method, be sure to pause appropriately.
■ Be certain to verify patient knowledge and understanding by asking questions that will tap her or his understanding of the information.

When greeting a patient, you may already have some information about the purpose for the visit. For instance, a receptionist may have noted a basic "complaint" or you might have documentation indicating why the patient has come to see you. During the greeting process, remember

1

that not only is it appropriate, but it is of utmost importance to ask, "What brings you in today?"

A critical aspect of meeting the needs of patients with hearing loss is to modify your style of interaction to facilitate optimal communication. For patients with known or suspected hearing loss, your speech should be slightly slower and slightly louder than normal and you should face the patient wherever possible. You should maintain your attention on the patient rather than on medical record-keeping or note-taking equipment. Most patients will have a limited understanding of the terminology formally used for describing anatomy of the auditory system and hearing function. It is important to modify your use of language to avoid jargon that will be confusing to the patient.

It is your responsibility to build rapport with patients so that they are comfortable with you. This will begin in the first few moments that you are with patients and will carry on throughout your relationship with them. In order to build rapport, you will need to possess and display genuine characteristics of objectivity, empathy, and respect. As a demonstration of the aforementioned characteristics, you also will need to convey a fundamental desire to listen in a sensitive manner.

Understanding the culture of patients you are greeting is critical. Patients from different cultural groups may respond to disability, eye contact, familial hierarchy, use of names and titles, and the role of different genders in society in a manner that is different from yours. You should be aware of these differences because they will set the stage for your interactions with the patient from the very beginning. When greeting patients, be sensitive to their cultural background. In general, follow these guidelines:

- Use a title such as "Mr." or "Ms."
- Ensure that you are talking with the correct person. Use at least two other identifiers, such as birth date and address, to confirm identity.
- Identify yourself and your purpose.
- If the patient is accompanied by another person, ask if this person should be present during the patient's examination.

Say, for example, "Hello Ms. Smith. My name is (state your title, and first and last name). I am the audiologist who will be testing your hearing today/seeing you today. Our appointment should take about (insert number of minutes). Can I have you confirm your (address, date of birth, identification number, phone number, other identifier) for me?"

## Explaining the Evaluation

After you have greeted the patient and confirmed her or his identity, explain the process of the evaluation. Say, for example, "First, I will be talking with you about what brings you in today. Then I will be looking in your ears, and testing your hearing. I also will be testing how well your eardrums and the bones in your middle ears are functioning. These tests will help me understand more about your hearing and any difficulties you might be having." This brief statement gives the patient a sense of the overall structure of the appointment. Then ask, "Do you have any questions before we begin?"

## OBSERVATION

1. Observe an experienced clinician greeting a patient.

2. Observe the elements that the clinician uses to build rapport.

    a. What specific behaviors does the clinician use?

    b. Does the clinician's choice of words appear appropriate for the patient's cognitive level, chronologic age, and hearing status?

3. If an interpreter is present, note how the clinician interacts with the patient and the interpreter.

    a. To whom does the clinician address her or his questions?

## GUIDED PRACTICE

1. Prepare to greet a patient on your own. Utilize demographic and other available information to learn about the patient prior to the visit.

2. Based on the information that you have, briefly list the assumptions that you are making prior to meeting with the patient.

    _I will assume something with their hearing is why they are coming in, so I would speak loudly and clearly._

3. Greet the patient. Remember to speak slowly and clearly.

4. Verify the patient's identity, and review the plan of action for the appointment with him or her.

5. Test any assumptions you have noted in item number 2.

6. Make certain that the patient is comfortable with the process and has an opportunity to ask questions.

## REFLECTION AND REVIEW

1. Describe in detail how you would greet a patient. Include the following:

   a. Addressing the patient

   b. Confirming the patient's identity

   c. Providing an overview of the activities of the appointment, as well as the time frame in which they will be conducted

   d. Asking the patient for any questions about the process

   _Hello, how are you today? I am Abby Rushford and I will be doing your exam today. What is your name and date of birth for confirmation? First we will talk about why you are here today, then I will take a look in you ears. Do you have any questions?_

2. What specific behaviors might you display to earn the patient's trust and respect?

   _I will be polite and be professionally dressed with my name tag._

3. Describe in detail the information you might obtain from preexisting demographic information, referral information, previous chart notes, and other patient information. How you would test any assumptions that you are making?

I would look over charts and past exams. Then I would do my own screening and compare / contrast. I would also see if the client's hearing has gotten better or if it has worsened.

4. Discuss how you would work with an interpreter during a visit. How would you verify patient understanding of the information you are sharing and discussing?

I would ask if the interpreter is interpreting sequentially or simultaneously. Then I would be sure to speak slowly and clearly. Lastly, I would speak directly to the patient.

# ┃┃┃2┃┃┃

## The Patient Interview

## INTRODUCTION

The patient interview is the first step of the audiologic assessment. Determining which tests to perform and why to perform them typically stems from information gathered during the interview process. The interview provides vital information regarding the patient's symptoms and history that help to understand testing outcomes. In this chapter, you will practice interviewing so that you will be prepared to uncover the issues impacting your patient.

## LEARNING OUTCOMES

■ Understand the purpose of obtaining a patient history.
■ Know what type of information to gather in the patient interview.
■ Be able to perform a patient interview.

## REVIEW OF CONCEPTS

### Greeting the Patient

The willingness of a patient to share historical and personal information involves a degree of confidence and trust in the clinician. Chapter 1 provided basic principles of greeting the patient and establishing rapport that will serve as the foundation for the history gathering process. Your ability to foster a constructive relationship with your patient will impact your success with gathering important information.

### Purpose of the Patient Interview

The purpose of the patient interview is to gain an understanding of the medical, social, educational, occupational, recreational, and developmental past of the patient to determine the issues relevant to the audiologic examination and to assist in interpretation of audiometric data and formulation of recommendations. Typically, initial visits require more data gathering from the patient; established patients may require less inquiry. The appointment type often will impact the amount of information gathered as well (e.g., a vestibular evaluation typically requires more extensive data gathering than a referral solely for tympanometry).

## Gathering Information

As you conduct the interview, there will be both patient and clinician responsibilities. The patient will be responsible for providing reliable and accurate information. The clinician has several responsibilities. First, the clinician must build rapport with the patient. Therefore, the clinician should look at the patient while conducting the interview, versus focusing on note taking. Second, the clinician should allow the conversation with the patient to flow naturally and request missing information as needed. The clinician must monitor the discussion and avoid asking the same questions repeatedly simply to follow the order of questions on a form. Third, the clinician must minimize discussion of factors that do not directly influence the case. Not all information will be relevant, and too much exploration of unrelated issues will be costly in terms of time. Although the content of complete audiologic case history documentation varies (either by clinician or facility preference), the main points are listed below.

## Basic Patient Information

- Patient demographic information
- Referral source
  - Physician or other provider
  - Self-referral
- Primary complaint
- Hearing loss
  - Ear specificity
  - Previous hearing evaluation
    - Changes in hearing over time
  - Onset of hearing loss
    - Congenital or acquired
    - Onset relative to speech and language development
    - Gradual or sudden

- Stability of hearing loss
  - Factors that the patient notices relevant to fluctuation or progression
- Impact of hearing loss on the patient's life
- Previous experience with hearing instruments and/or assistive listening devices
  - Current and past hearing instrument use
  - Interest in hearing instrument use
- Family history of hearing loss
- Exposure to loud noise
  - Type of noise
  - Duration of exposure
  - Time since last exposure to noise
- Pain, fullness, or pressure in the ears
  - Ear specificity
  - Current presence of symptom
  - Occurrence and duration of last episode of symptom
  - Related reduction in hearing sensitivity
- Experience with otitis media or otitis externa
  - Dates of occurrence
  - Previous treatment
  - Drainage
- History of previous ear surgeries
  - Ear specificity
  - Type of surgery
  - Date of surgery
- Tinnitus
  - Ear specificity
  - Description of sensation
  - Impact on the patient
- Dizziness
  - Description of sensation
  - Nausea/vomiting
  - Activities that precipitate dizziness
  - Occurrence and duration of dizziness
  - Factors that cause a reduction of symptoms
  - Other symptoms observed with the dizziness
- Current medications (prescription and over the counter)
  - Use of other substances (other drugs, alcohol, caffeine, etc.)
- Other medical problems

## Pediatric Patient Interview

When working with children and the parents or guardians of children, many of the same basic questions will apply. However, these questions may be framed differently and must be considered in the context of the child's overall development. Some additional areas of exploration are noted here:

- Concerns about hearing
- Overall development
  - Global or specific delays
  - Age of standing, crawling, walking
  - Age of potty-training
  - Fine motor skill acquisition
- Speech and language development, including preliteracy skills
  - Age of first word
  - Age of two-word combinations
  - Use of gesture/other nonverbal cues
  - Overall intelligibility and complexity of child's speech utterances
  - History of speech and language screening or evaluation
  - Services for speech-language pathology or other rehabilitation or intervention
- Pregnancy, birth, and postnatal history
  - Unusual problems during birth
  - Exposure to viral disease during pregnancy
  - Medications/drugs/alcohol used during the pregnancy
  - Child's birth weight
  - Time spent in intensive care nursery
  - Family history of hearing loss
  - Presence of craniofacial anomalies
- Otologic history
  - History of fluid in ears
  - History of ventilation tubes
  - Date of most recent ear infection
  - Current medications
- Audiologic intervention
  - Use of hearing instruments or cochlear implant
    - Duration of use
    - Success with device(s)
- Educational and social functioning

## OBSERVATION

1. Observe an experienced clinician conduct a patient interview.

2. Observe the elements that the clinician uses to build rapport.

   a. What specific behaviors does the clinician use?

   b. Does the clinician's choice of words appear appropriate for the patient's cognitive level, chronologic age, and hearing status?

3. Observe the tools that the clinician uses to conduct the interview.

   a. Is the interview initiated by having the patient complete a case history form?

   b. Does the clinician use the patient's paperwork for further notation, or does the clinician have a separate form or electronic system?

   c. Where is the clinician's focus during the interview—on the patient or on the tools?

4. Observe how the clinician guides the conversation depending on the answers given by the patient.

   a. Does the clinician ask for clarification or repetition?

   b. Does the clinician always follow the same format, or does the clinician follow the patient's lead?

## GUIDED PRACTICE

1. Develop your own instrument to capture the patient history information.

2. Prepare to gather a patient history on your own. Verify as much information about the patient as you can before the visit through any paperwork.

3. Think of ways to be flexible during the interview.

   a. How/when will you ask probing questions?

   b. What can you do to avoid asking the same question more than once?

   c. How will you stay on task?

4. Obtain an understanding of why the patient is being evaluated by asking the patient the reason for the visit.

5. Perform a patient interview including the components described above.

## REFLECTION AND REVIEW

1. The act of greeting the patient and building rapport is described in Chapter 1. Explain why this is important prior to initiating a patient interview.

   _This is important to build trust so that the client will be confident and share all needed information_

2. How might the information gathered in the patient interview assist in the interpretation of the audiologic testing outcomes?

   _The info from the interview will give us an idea of what is going on before looking at the test results_

3. Explain why questioning the patient regarding hearing loss may be helpful prior to performing audiologic testing.

    This will help us determine how long the issue has lasted and the severity

4. Provide reasons why patient report of tinnitus perception may be important in interpreting diagnostic results.

    This will tell us the issue is located in the ear and can lead us to a diagnosis

5. Explain how symptoms of pain, pressure, or fullness might be related to audiologic testing outcomes.

    It presents a current symptom

6. Explain why a history of ear surgery is important to know prior to audiologic assessment.

    This surgery may have affected hearing loss

7. Explain why use of medications and/or drugs should be explored.

    The meds may be causing the hearing loss or worsening it

8. Explain why patient reports of dizziness should be described in detail.

    The occurance of the dizzyness can help us find a diagnosis

9. Explain why history of noise exposure might be important in the interpretation of audiologic outcomes. Why are the details of the noise exposure also important?

The hearing loss may be noise induced from working in a loud place or from concerts, etc.

# ‖‖ 3 ‖‖

## Otoscopic Examination

Observation of the status of the ear canal and tympanic membrane provides information regarding potential concerns for conductive hearing loss. It is necessary to assess the ear canal prior to performing audiologic tests to determine the safety of performing such measures and to assist in interpretation of audiologic results.

## LEARNING OUTCOMES

- Understand the purpose of the otoscopic examination.
- Be able to perform an otoscopic examination using a handheld otoscope.
- Be able to identify landmarks of the tympanic membrane when performing otoscopy.
- Be able to identify cerumen and determine the need for cerumen removal prior to performing audiologic testing.
- Know what signs may indicate middle ear or external ear canal pathology.

## REVIEW OF CONCEPTS

There are several reasons to perform an otoscopic examination at each evaluation and treatment session. The audiologist must visualize the external ear canal and tympanic membrane to understand the physical influences that can impact the outcome of the audiologic evaluation. It is necessary to determine that it is safe to perform audiologic testing involving the placement of probe tips and earphones into the ear canal. The presence of foreign bodies or cerumen in the ear canal has the potential to impact immittance measures and to create a conductive hearing loss. Observation of the tympanic membrane allows the clinician to have insight, prior to testing, regarding pathology or structural differences that may impact test results.

### Collapsed Ear Canal

The ear canal itself must be observed prior to testing. In some patients, the cartilage of the ear canal is quite pliable. The use of supra-aural earphones in such a case can actually collapse the ear canal, resulting in a conductive hearing loss due to attenuation of sound. This phenomenon generally can be remedied by the use of insert earphones to obtain a valid assessment of hearing.

## Performing Otoscopy

An otoscopic examination typically is performed using a handheld otoscope. The otoscope has a light source that must be turned on prior to use. The otoscope contains lenses, which magnify the image of the ear canal. A speculum is placed on the end of the otoscope and is placed into the ear canal. The audiologist can visualize the components of the ear canal and tympanic membrane by looking through the viewing window of the otoscope.

To perform otoscopy, the otoscope is held in one hand, near the "head" of the otoscope. Using the other hand, the pinna is gently pulled up and toward the back of the patient's head to straighten out the normally "S-shaped" ear canal and allow for visualization of the tympanic membrane. The tip of the speculum of the otoscope is gently advanced into the external ear canal as shown in

Figure 3–1. Importantly, the fingers of the hand holding the otoscope are placed against the head of the patient. By doing this, the otoscope will be unable to move independently of the patient's head. This is important, so that if the patient moves during the examination, the otoscope tip will not cause damage to the patient's ear canal. The patient should be instructed to remain still during the otoscopic examination to allow for visualization and to prevent injury to the ear canal.

## Landmarks

In the case of a normal ear canal and tympanic membrane, there are a number of landmarks to be visualized. A drawing of the tympanic membrane is shown in Figure 3–2.

The "light reflex" or "cone of light" is a reflection of the light source used for otoscopy that appears in the inferior anterior quadrant of the normal tympanic membrane. The cone of light can be used as a landmark to orient the viewer. The presence of the cone of light also is an indication of a normally shaped, concave tympanic membrane

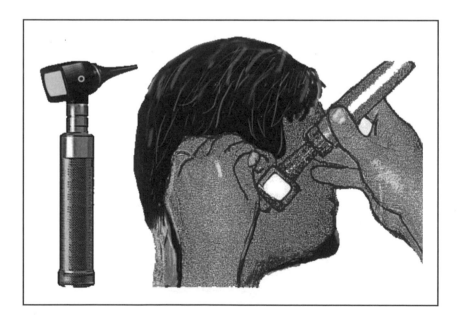

**FIGURE 3–1.** Otoscopic examination using a handheld otoscope. (Source unknown. From *Basics of Audiology: From Vibration to Sound*, by J. L. Cranford. Copyright © 2007 Plural Publishing, Inc. All rights reserved. Used with permission.)

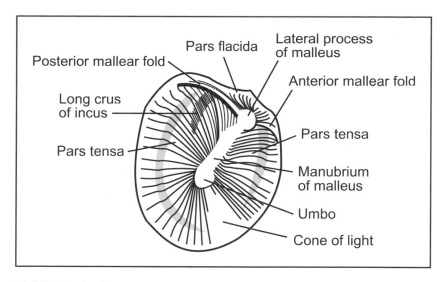

**FIGURE 3–2.** Tympanic membrane. (From *Otolaryngology Head and Neck Surgery: Clinical Reference Guide* [2nd ed.], by R. Pasha. Copyright © 2006 Plural Publishing, Inc. All rights reserved. Used with permission.)

—that is, the tympanic membrane is neither "bulging," as in the case of an otitis media, nor retracted.

The annulus, the ring of cartilage surrounding the tympanic membrane, also may be visualized. At the top of the tympanic membrane, an area of reduced tension, known as the *pars flaccida*, may be seen.

The normal tympanic membrane has a concave shape. This is due to the attachment of the middle of the tympanic membrane to the manubrium of the malleus, known as the *umbo*. Depending on the thickness of the tympanic membrane, some other structures of the middle ear space may be visualized, including the long process of the incus, and/or the stapedial tendon. A normal tympanic membrane is shown in Figure 3–3.

## Cerumen

The presence of cerumen in an ear canal is a normal and healthy phenomenon. Cerumen varies in appearance, depending on its consistency. Cerumen most often is a yellowish or brownish color, and may appear to be hard or soft. Typically, the

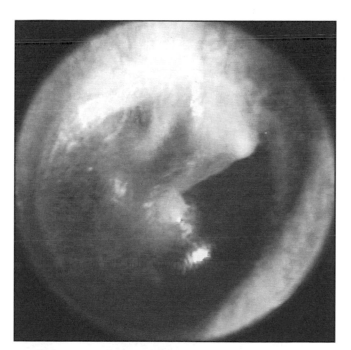

**FIGURE 3–3.** Normal tympanic membrane. The cone of light can be visualized in the inferior anterior quadrant. The umbo can be visualized in the center of tympanic membrane. (From *Atlas of Otoscopy*, by J. Touma and B. Touma. Copyright © 2006 Plural Publishing, Inc. All rights reserved. Used with permission.)

presence of excessive cerumen creates a high-frequency hearing loss. When cerumen completely occludes the ear canal, a flat conductive hearing loss may be found. In cases where cerumen has the potential to influence audiologic outcomes, it should be removed prior to initiation of testing.

## Foreign Bodies

Any variety of foreign bodies may be present in the ear canal including cotton swabs or tissue, insects, pieces of hearing aids such as wax traps or open-ear domes, or any other objects that fit inside the ear canal. In Figure 3–4, an insect can be seen in the ear canal.

## Exostoses

Exostoses are bony growths in the ear canal. In most cases, these growths are harmless. Location and size must be noted to determine whether there

is potential for interference with earphone placement and, therefore, with audiometric outcomes. An example of exostoses can be seen in Figure 3–5.

## Tympanosclerosis

Calcifications may occur on the tympanic membrane as a result of inflammation of the membrane. This condition, known as *tympanosclerosis*, results in white, generally horseshoe-shaped marks on the tympanic membrane.

## Perforations

A perforation of the tympanic membrane may allow visualization of the middle ear structures. An example of a perforation of the tympanic membrane is shown in Figure 3–6. In some cases, a very thin layer of tympanic membrane may form following previous perforation. This neomembrane often is mistaken for a current perforation.

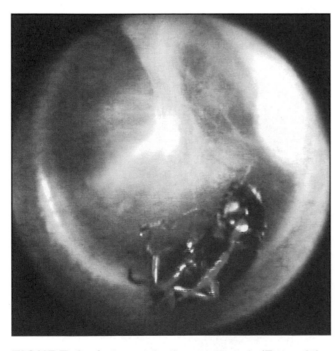

**FIGURE 3–4.** Insect in the ear canal. (From *Atlas of Otoscopy*, by J. Touma and B. Touma. Copyright © 2006 Plural Publishing, Inc. All rights reserved. Used with permission.)

**FIGURE 3–5.** Exostoses of the ear canal. (From *Atlas of Otoscopy*, by J. Touma and B. Touma. Copyright © 2006 Plural Publishing, Inc. All rights reserved. Used with permission.)

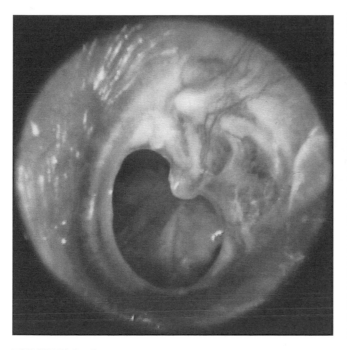

**FIGURE 3–6.** Perforation of the tympanic membrane. (From *Atlas of Otoscopy*, by J. Touma and B. Touma. Copyright © 2006 Plural Publishing, Inc. All rights reserved. Used with permission.)

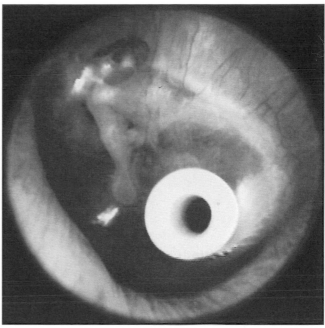

**FIGURE 3–7.** Pressure equalization tube in situ in the tympanic membrane. (From *Atlas of Otoscopy*, by J. Touma and B. Touma. Copyright © 2006 Plural Publishing, Inc. All rights reserved. Used with permission.)

## Pressure Equalization Tubes

Pressure equalization tubes are surgically placed in the tympanic membrane in cases of eustachian tube dysfunction. An example of a pressure equalization tube in the tympanic membrane is shown in Figure 3–7. If the tube is in place, it is important to note whether the tube appears patent or if wax or other debris appears to be blocking the opening of the tube. In some cases, the tube may be partially extruded from the tympanic membrane, may be found in the ear canal, or, very rarely, may be visualized in the middle ear space.

## Otitis Media

In the case of otitis media, various anomalies of the tympanic membrane can be seen. When excessive fluid is present in the middle ear space, a bulging tympanic membrane may be observed. An example of a bulging tympanic membrane is shown in Figure 3–8.

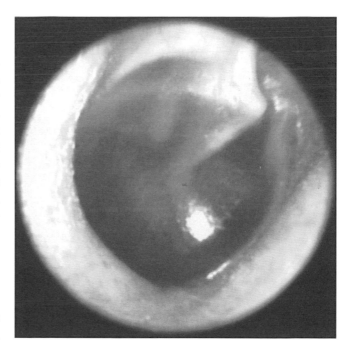

**FIGURE 3–8.** Bulging tympanic membrane due to otitis media. (From *Atlas of Otoscopy*, by J. Touma and B. Touma. Copyright © 2006 Plural Publishing, Inc. All rights reserved. Used with permission.)

In other phases of otitis media, air bubbles or a fluid line may be observed through the tympanic membrane. An example of air bubbles visualized through the tympanic membrane is shown in Figure 3–9.

In some cases, the tympanic membrane may appear to be retracted against the handle of the malleus or other structures of the middle ear space. In Figure 3–10, the tympanic membrane is retracted over the malleus.

## External Otitis

External otitis is an inflammation of the external ear canal. Other external ear canal conditions can be visualized during otoscopy, such as growth of fungus.

## When to Refer

Otoscopic examination of the ear canal may reveal situations or conditions that require referral to a medical physician for treatment. Such conditions include, but are not limited to, bleeding or discharge from the ear, evidence of infection in the middle ear space or ear canal, evidence of fluid in the middle ear space, perforation of the tympanic membrane, presence of foreign objects in the ear canal, visible ear canal obstruction or abnormalities, and cerumen that is deep in the ear canal or of a consistency that cannot be removed without risk of damage to the ear canal.

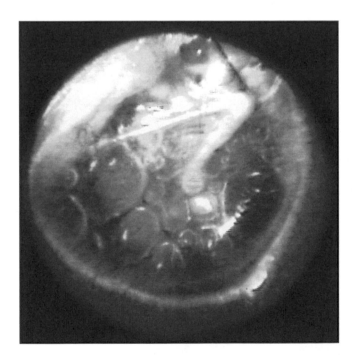

**FIGURE 3–9.** Air bubbles visualized behind tympanic membrane. (From *Atlas of Otoscopy*, by J. Touma and B. Touma. Copyright © 2006 Plural Publishing, Inc. All rights reserved. Used with permission.)

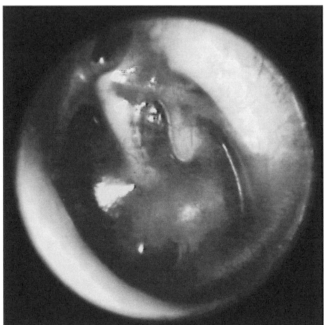

**FIGURE 3–10.** Retracted tympanic membrane. (From *Atlas of Otoscopy*, by J. Touma and B. Touma. Copyright © 2006 Plural Publishing, Inc. All rights reserved. Used with permission.)

## OBSERVATION

1. Observe an experienced clinician using an otoscope to perform an otoscopic examination. Carefully observe the clinician's method of bracing the otoscope to prevent injury.

2. If available, observe a clinician utilizing a video otoscope to perform an otoscopic examination. Observe the landmarks of the ear canal and tympanic membrane.

3. Listen carefully to how the audiologist describes her or his findings of otoscopy to the patient. What terms does the audiologist use in describing the findings?

## GUIDED PRACTICE

1. Perform an otoscopic examination on a patient using an otoscope. Ensure that the otoscope is braced properly for examination.

2. Describe the ear canal and tympanic membrane that you view. Identify the cone of light, the annulus, and the umbo.

## REFLECTION AND REVIEW

1. Sketch an image of a normal tympanic membrane and label the following landmarks: light reflex, annulus, pars flaccida, and umbo. Is your image of a left or right tympanic membrane? How can you tell?

1. right ear
2. by the way the cone of light reflects

pars flaccida

annulus

umbo

cone of light

2. What is the concern regarding audiologic outcomes in the case of a collapsed ear canal? What strategy can be used to prevent a collapsed ear canal?

A collapsed ear canal can result in conductive hearing loss. To prevent this use insert earphones to get a valid assessment.

3. After performing an otoscopic examination, describe how the otoscope was braced against the head of the patient.

You place your other hand on their head to stabilize and prevent injury

4. List three otoscopic findings that might lead to a physician referral.

Referral is needed when there is bleeding/discharge, infection, and fluid in middle ear

5. Write a description of normal otoscopic findings. Use terminology that you would use when describing this to a patient.

You will be able to visualize the cone of light, the annulus, and the ear drum should have a concave shape.

6. How do the results of otoscopy impact the clinician's assumptions and testing procedures for audiometry and immittance testing?

The results will show if there is an issue or problem that need further testing or procedures

# ║║║ 4 ║║║

## Immittance Instrumentation

### INTRODUCTION

The immittance meter is a tool that allows inference of aspects of auditory system function. In this chapter, you will explore your immittance meter and become familiar and comfortable with its use. This chapter reviews the characteristics of the equipment. Review of concepts regarding immittance testing procedures and results of immittance testing are addressed in Chapters 5, 6, and 7.

*Note:* Every style and model of immittance instrument is different. There may be controls and options addressed in this chapter that are not available on the machine you are using. Nevertheless, it is important to understand these functions, as you may encounter them on equipment in the future. Alternatively, the equipment that you are using may have features and functions that are not addressed in this chapter. The authors encourage you to become familiar with these features and functions as well. The user manual for your particular equipment is a helpful tool for understanding the various components of your immittance machine.

### LEARNING OUTCOMES

■ Know the fundamental components of the immittance instrumentation.
■ Know the types of tests available on the immittance instrumentation you are using.
■ Know the ranges of the various parameters of the immittance instrumentation you are using.
■ Become comfortable with manipulation of controls on the immittance meter.
■ Be able to manipulate controls to present desired stimuli.

### REVIEW OF CONCEPTS

#### What Is an Immittance Meter?

An immittance meter is a device used to make measures to infer auditory system function including tympanometry, acoustic reflex threshold, and acoustic reflex decay. The device relies on principles of immittance that are described in the following chapters.

The immittance meter has an air pump and manometer to alter and measure pressure in the ear canal. It also has a probe tone generator and a transducer that delivers the tone into the external ear canal. A microphone is also located in the probe unit that fits into the ear canal. A schematic of the probe is shown in Figure 4–1.

The instrument functions by measuring the sound pressure level (SPL) of the probe tone, providing information about the admittance of energy into the middle ear space, from which inferences are made about the functionality of the middle ear system. The immittance instrument also is capable of delivering additional stimuli that are used to activate a muscle response in the middle ear system. This acoustic reflex response is addressed in Chapters 6 and 7.

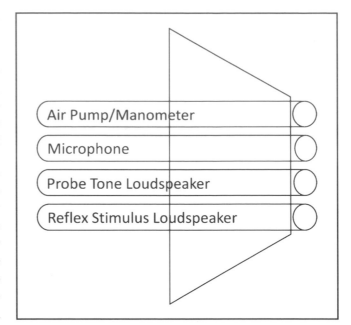

**FIGURE 4–1.** Immittance probe.

## Display and Control Panels

The control panel contains a variety of controls that are used to manipulate the test parameters and stimulus characteristics. The test parameters include the type of test to be performed, as well as the characteristics of the measurement. For example, you can choose to perform tympanometry (type of test), a diagnostic test versus a screening test (type of test), the rate of pressure change for the recording of the tympanogram (test parameter), and the range of pressure variation for the recording of the tympanogram (test parameter). The ear to which you present the stimulus is a test parameter as well, and it may be selected for recording on certain machines. In addition to test parameters, stimulus characteristics can be manipulated. Examples of these characteristics are the type of stimulus (pure tone versus noise), the frequency of the stimulus, and the intensity of the stimulus. For example, when performing an acoustic reflex threshold test, it may be specified that a 1000 Hz pure tone is presented at 95 dB SPL.

The display panel of the immittance meter reflects the test parameters and stimulus characteristics chosen for testing. This panel also displays the results of the testing performed.

## GUIDED PRACTICE

Perform these immittance measures with a volunteer. Perform the test on another person and then have the test performed on you.

1. Find the power switch for the immittance instrument, and turn it on.

2. What is the make and model of the immittance machine that you are using?

_____

3. On what date was the machine last calibrated?

_____

4. Identify where the outputs for the machine are located.

5. Examine the probe. How many ports are there, and what do they do?

_____

_____

6. Identify the controls for the immittance meter. Determine the specific controls for types of tests, stimulus, intensity, and test start.

7. Set the equipment to perform tympanometry. Set the probe tone to 226 Hz. Examine the display screen. What is the range of pressure variation in the ear canal that can be generated?

_____

8. Obtain a seal with the probe in the ear canal, and run a tympanogram. This will require you to select a probe tip that will fit snugly into the opening of your volunteer's ear canal. Be patient with this process, using gentle pressure to fit the probe tip into the canal opening. Press the appropriate button to start the test. Observe the response.

9. Change the type of test to a screening mode if available. Insert the probe into the ear canal, and obtain a seal. What happens?

_____

10. Return to a diagnostic mode. Determine whether the frequency of the probe tone can be changed on your equipment. If so, what other frequency options are available?

_____

11. Examine the display screen. Identify the location of the measurements for equivalent ear canal volume, tympanometric peak pressure, tympanometric static admittance, and tympanometric width.

12. Are there alternative settings for the rate of pressure change? If so, what are the options?

_____

13. Are there alternative settings for the starting pressure level? If so, what are the options?

_____

14. Is there a rotary knob on the immittance machine? What is the purpose of the knob?

_____

_____

15. Change the test type to acoustic reflex threshold measurement.

16. Identify the contralateral stimulus earphone. Place this into the contralateral ear canal with the appropriate probe tip.

17. Review the options available for stimulus type. What options are available?

_____

_____

_____

18. Review the options available for stimulus intensity. What are the ranges available for each stimulus type?

_____

_____

_____

_____

_____

_____

19. Obtain a seal with the probe in the ipsilateral ear canal. Begin the acoustic reflex test by pressurizing the ear canal. Set the stimulus to deliver a 1000 Hz tone at 80 dB SPL to the ipsilateral ear. Use the presentation button to deliver the stimulus. Observe the response.

20. Change the stimulus to deliver a 2000 Hz tone to the contralateral ear at 90 dB SPL. Use the presentation button to deliver the stimulus. Observe the response.

21. Change the test type to acoustic reflex decay measurement.

22. Set the stimulus to deliver a 1000 Hz tone at 95 dB SPL to the contralateral ear. Use the start button to begin the stimulus. Observe the response.

23. Review the manufacturer's directions for cleaning and maintaining the probe and tubes. Practice this using the equipment provided by the manufacturer.

24. Determine whether there is a calibration check unit. Review the manufacturer's directions for a calibration check of the unit, and perform a calibration check.

## REFLECTION AND REVIEW

1. If the tubing on the end of the probe unit were to be damaged, would it be appropriate to cut the length of the tubing? Why or why not?

   _no, because the tubing could be too short to get an accurate test reading._

2. What controls and options are available on the immittance machine in your clinic that are not discussed in this chapter?

   _The controls/options are very similar to the ones in our clinic._

# ‖‖5‖‖

## Tympanometry

## INTRODUCTION

Tympanometry is an essential component of the audiologic evaluation. Use of tympanometry allows the clinician to have an objective measure that contributes to the understanding of middle ear function.

## LEARNING OUTCOMES

■ Understand the purpose of tympanometry.
■ Know how to obtain a tympanogram.
■ Understand how to interpret a tympanogram.

## REVIEW OF CONCEPTS

Admittance is a measure of the ease with which sound energy is transferred into the middle ear space. Tympanometry involves measuring admittance while varying pressure in the ear canal relative to atmospheric pressure. When the eustachian tube is functioning properly, the air trapped in the middle ear space tends to be maintained at atmospheric pressure. When the middle ear system is functioning optimally, the greatest admittance of sound energy into the middle ear system occurs at atmospheric pressure. When there is pathology that disturbs function of the eustachian tube, the greatest admittance of sound energy into the middle ear system may occur at a different pressure level (positive relative to atmospheric pressure, or more commonly, negative relative to atmospheric pressure). In some cases, for example when the middle ear is filled with fluid, there is little admittance of sound energy into the middle ear system. These effects can be observed on the tympanogram.

### Tympanometric Measurement

To perform tympanometry, an immittance probe is inserted into the opening of the ear canal. An airtight seal must be obtained in order to vary pressure in the ear canal. The immittance meter probe has an air pump to adjust air pressure in the ear canal, a manometer to measure air pressure, a microphone to measure the intensity of sound in the ear canal, and a loudspeaker to deliver a probe tone. A schematic of a probe unit with the components necessary for tympanometry is shown in Figure 5–1.

In order to measure immittance, a probe tone is presented continuously to maintain a fixed intensity level in the ear canal. The probe tone most commonly used for adults is 226 Hz, and for infants, 1000 Hz. As the probe tone is being presented, some of the sound energy is entering the middle ear system, and some of the sound energy is being maintained in the ear canal. The total sound energy in the ear canal is measured with the microphone. A schematic of this process is shown in Figure 5–2.

The amount of sound energy admitted to the middle ear system is related to the air pressure on either side of the tympanic membrane. When sound energy is transferred from one area to another where the air pressures are relatively equal, much of the energy is admitted into the next area. So, when the air pressure is equal on both sides of the tympanic membrane, the sound energy most easily travels into the middle ear space, and the sound pressure level (SPL) in the ear canal becomes lower. A schematic of this scenario is shown in Figure 5–3.

Alternatively, when pressure in the ear canal is greater than or less than the pressure in the middle ear space, less sound energy is transferred. Compared to an equal pressure condition, much more sound energy is maintained in the ear canal, resulting in a higher SPL. A schematic of this scenario is shown in Figure 5–4.

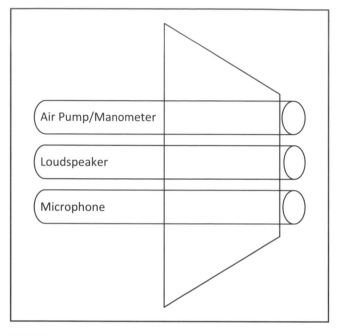

**FIGURE 5–1.** Immittance probe unit for tympanometry.

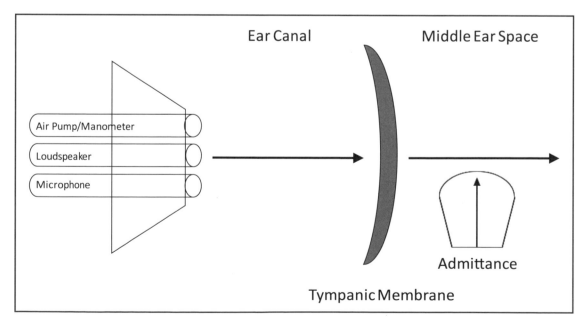

**FIGURE 5–2.** Admittance of sound energy. The probe tone is emitted by the loudspeaker in the probe unit. Some sound energy is transferred to the middle ear space. Some sound energy remains in the ear canal. The energy of the remaining sound is measured by the microphone located in the probe unit.

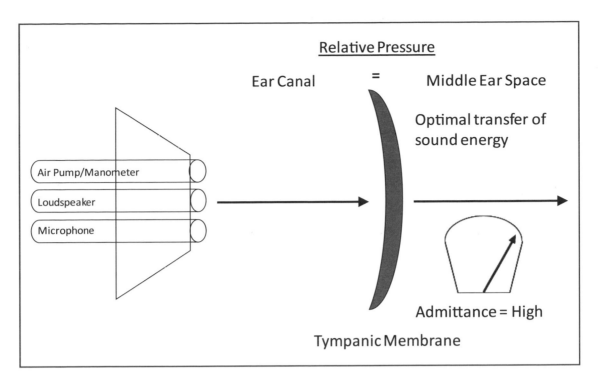

**FIGURE 5–3.** Optimal transfer of sound energy. The pressure is equal on both sides of the tympanic membrane, resulting in optimal transfer of sound energy through the tympanic membrane.

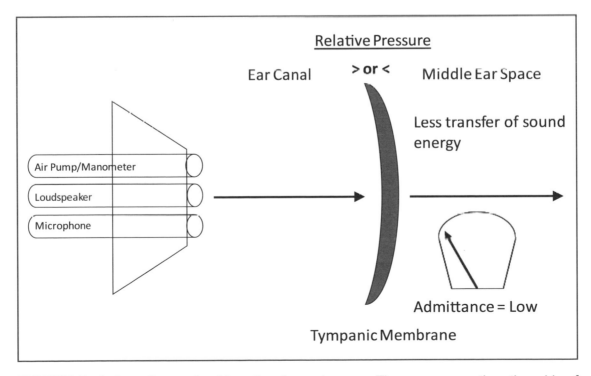

**FIGURE 5–4.** Less than optimal transfer of sound energy. The pressure on the other side of the tympanic membrane (in the middle ear space) is different than from that in the ear canal. Compared to a condition of equal pressure, less sound energy is transferred through the tympanic membrane, and more sound energy remains in the ear canal.

The process for measurement of the admitted sound energy to the middle ear space can be conceptualized as follows. When performing tympanometry, the loudspeaker delivers a probe tone of known intensity into the ear canal. The microphone picks up the remaining auditory signal. A device known as an automatic gain control compares the difference in the electrical signal for the loudspeaker and the microphone and continuously adjusts the level of the probe tone coming from the loudspeaker so that the sound pressure level in the ear canal remains constant. By comparing the difference between the amplified probe tone signal and the sound pressure level picked up by the microphone, it can be determined how much sound energy was admitted into the middle ear space. A schematic of this process is shown in Figure 5–5. Admittance of sound pressure into the middle ear space is measured in units of millimhos (mmho), millimeters of water (mm H$_2$O), or milliliters (mL).

While this sound measurement process is occurring, the air pump works to make a very positive pressure in the ear canal space. Then, the air pressure is decreased until the pressure is very negative in the ear canal space. (Alternatively, pressure may be increased from negative to positive). A schematic of this process is shown in Figure 5–6. By doing this, the admittance of sound energy into the middle ear space can be measured over a wide range of air pressures. Air pressure in the ear canal is measured in decapascals (daPa). The range of pressures measured on most tympanometers is approximately −400 daPa to +200 daPa, as shown in Figure 5–7.

The tympanogram is a graph of admittance of sound energy as a function of sound pressure in the ear canal. The air pressure is plotted on the abscissa. The admittance (in mmho, mm H$_2$O, or mL) is plotted on the ordinate. This graph is shown in Figure 5–8.

By introducing substantially positive pressure (+200 daPa) into the ear canal, the tympanic membrane and ossicular chain essentially become rigid structures. Very little admittance of sound energy into the middle ear space occurs. In the case of a normally functioning middle ear space, as the pressure is continuously decreased, a greater amount of sound energy is admitted into the middle ear space. Eventually, when the pressure in the ear canal equals the pressure in the middle ear space, the amount of admitted sound energy reaches a peak level. Then, as the pressure in the ear canal becomes negative relative to the pressure in the middle ear space, the admittance of sound energy into the middle ear space begins

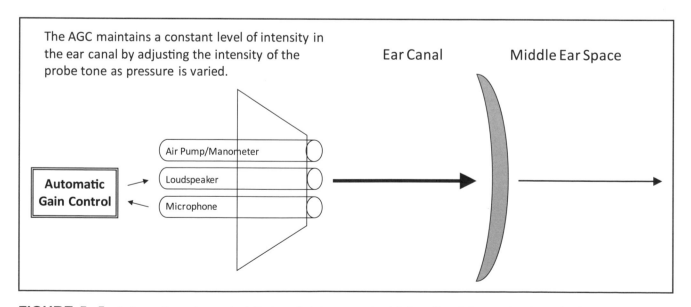

**FIGURE 5–5.** Automatic gain control that maintains constant intensity of the probe tone in the ear canal as pressure is varied.

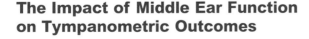

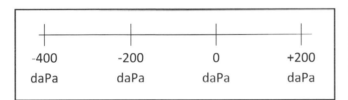

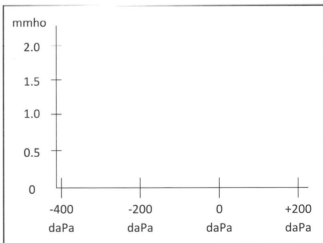

**FIGURE 5–6.** Air pump/manometer function. The air pump is used to vary the pressure of the ear canal space over time. The resulting changes in sound pressure level are reflected in the energy reaching the microphone of the probe unit.

**FIGURE 5–7.** Range of ear canal pressure generated by the air pump.

to decrease. We expect that when the middle ear is functioning optimally, the greatest amount of admittance will occur at about atmospheric pressure (0 daPa on the tympanogram). A tympanogram showing the greatest admittance occurring at 0 daPa is shown in Figure 5–9.

## The Impact of Middle Ear Function on Tympanometric Outcomes

Middle ear pathology often causes changes to the function of the admittance of sound energy to the middle ear system. Typically, the result is that there is less admittance of sound energy into the middle ear space under normal atmospheric

**FIGURE 5–8.** Graph axes comprising the tympanogram. The tympanogram is a graph of admittance of sound energy as a function of air pressure in the ear canal. The air pressure is plotted on the abscissa. The admittance (in mmho, mm $H_2O$, or mL) is plotted on the ordinate.

conditions. For example, at the onset or offset of otitis media, the pathophysiology of the condition often creates a situation where there is significant negative pressure in the middle ear space.

As mentioned previously, the greatest amount of admittance of sound energy to the middle ear system occurs when the pressure on either side of the tympanic membrane is relatively equal. When significant negative pressure exists in the middle ear space, then the greatest admittance will occur when the pressure in the ear canal is significantly negative. A tympanogram showing the greatest admittance occurring at a negative pressure of about −200 daPa is shown in Figure 5–10.

In cases of active otitis media, fluid may fill the middle ear space. In this case, there is very little admittance of sound energy into the middle ear space, regardless of the ear canal pressure. A schematic showing this process is shown in Figure 5–11. Because there is very little difference in the amount

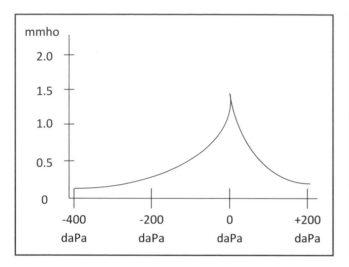

**FIGURE 5–9.** Tympanogram with peak admittance at 0 daPa.

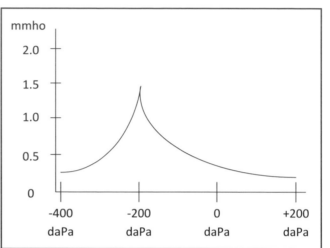

**FIGURE 5–10.** Tympanogram with peak admittance at −200 daPa, reflecting negative pressure in the middle ear space relative to pressure in the ear canal.

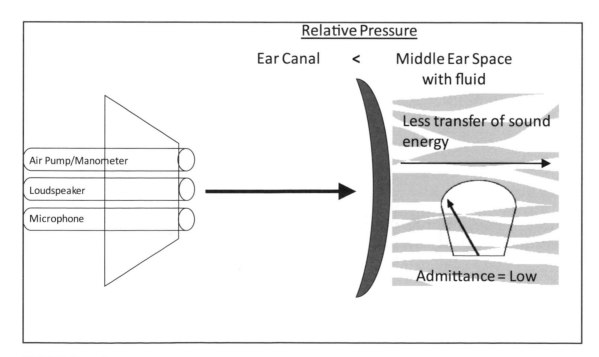

**FIGURE 5–11.** Effect of fluid in middle ear space on admittance of sound energy.

of admittance at any pressure level, the resulting graph appears to be relatively flat. The resulting tympanogram is shown in Figure 5–12.

The type of tympanometry described above is known as single-frequency tympanometry. There are other types of tympanometry, but single frequency is currently the most commonly used clinically.

## Measures Obtained for Single-Frequency Tympanometry

### *Tympanometric Static Admittance*

Tympanometric static admittance is determined by the height of the peak on the tympanogram. This measure is an indication of the amount of admittance of sound energy into the middle ear space. A schematic demonstrating measurement of this value from the tympanogram is shown in Figure 5–13.

### *Tympanometric Peak Pressure*

Tympanometric peak pressure is the pressure level at which the peak of the tympanogram occurs. This measure is an indication of the pressure level

at which the greatest admittance of sound energy occurs. From this, we can infer whether the pressure in the middle ear space is positive or negative relative to the pressure in the ear canal. A schematic demonstrating measurement of this value from the tympanogram is shown in Figure 5–14.

### *Tympanometric Width*

Tympanometric width is a measure of the width of the tympanogram measured at half of the static admittance from the peak to the admittance at +200 daPa. Certain pathologies, such as fluid

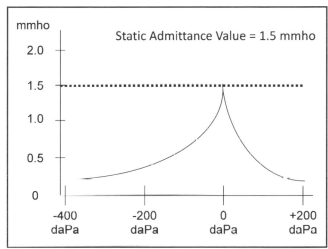

**FIGURE 5–13.** Measurement of tympanometric static admittance.

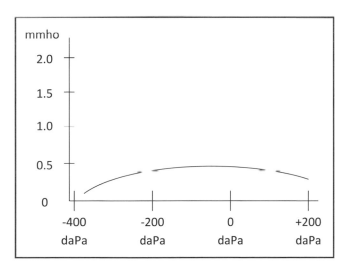

**FIGURE 5–12.** Tympanogram with no peak admittance. The presence of fluid in the middle ear space effectively creates a rigid tympanic membrane. The air-pressure changes introduced by the air pump do not cause a change in the compliance of the tympanic membrane or the admittance of sound energy into the middle ear space.

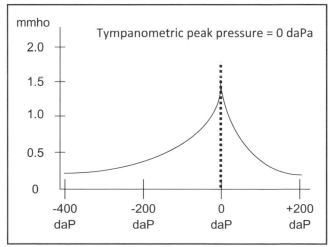

**FIGURE 5–14.** Measurement of tympanometric peak pressure.

in the middle ear, can increase tympanometric width. A schematic demonstrating this measurement is shown in Figure 5–15.

### Equivalent Ear Canal Volume

Equivalent ear canal volume is a measurement of the volume of air in front of the probe in cubic centimeters (cc) or milliliters (mL) when the ear canal is pressurized to +200 daPa. A schematic of this measurement process is shown in Figure 5–16.

In most adult cases where there is an intact tympanic membrane, the volume of air in the ear canal in front of the probe is around 1.0 cc. In children and infants it is typically smaller. This measurement is useful for determining whether there

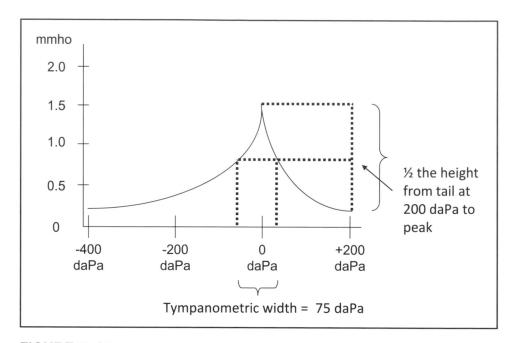

**FIGURE 5–15.** Measurement of tympanometric width.

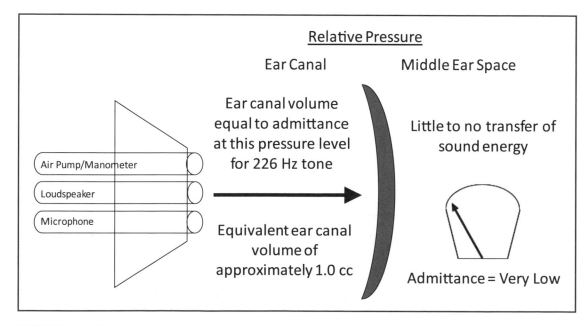

**FIGURE 5–16.** Measurement process of equivalent ear canal volume.

is an opening in the tympanic membrane (either due to perforation or to patent pressure equalization tubes), which allows measurement of the entire ear canal and middle ear system, demonstrated by an abnormally large volume. Typically, when this is the case, the tympanogram shape is flat or otherwise abnormal. A schematic demonstrating measurement of a large volume of air due to a tympanic membrane perforation is shown in Figure 5–17.

### Tympanometric Shape

The shape, a combination of the height and location of the tympanometric peak, has long been used to describe the tympanogram. The typically used shape types are as follows:

*Type A: Normal peak height and normal peak pressure.* A schematic demonstrating a Type A tympanogram is shown in Figure 5–18A.

*Type B: Flat.* This type of tympanogram is typically seen with middle ear dysfunction characterized by the addition of mass to the system, such as fluid behind the tympanic membrane. This type can also occur in the presence of ceru-

men impaction. A schematic demonstrating a Type B tympanogram is shown in Figure 5–18B.

*Type C: Negative peak pressure.* This type of tympanogram typically is seen with eustachian tube dysfunction. A schematic demonstrating a Type C tympanogram is shown in Figure 5–18C.

*Type $A_s$: Abnormally low peak height and normal peak pressure.* This type of tympanogram is consistent with an increase in the stiffness of the middle ear mechanism. A schematic demonstrating a Type $A_s$ tympanogram, often seen in disorders such as otosclerosis, is shown in Figure 5–18D.

*Type $A_d$: Abnormally high peak height and normal peak pressure.* This type of tympanogram is consistent with a decrease in the stiffness of the middle ear mechanism. A schematic demonstrating a Type $A_d$ tympanogram, often seen in ossicular disarticulation, is shown in Figure 5–18E.

### Performing Tympanometry

To perform tympanometry, the patient should be instructed to sit quietly and should be told what

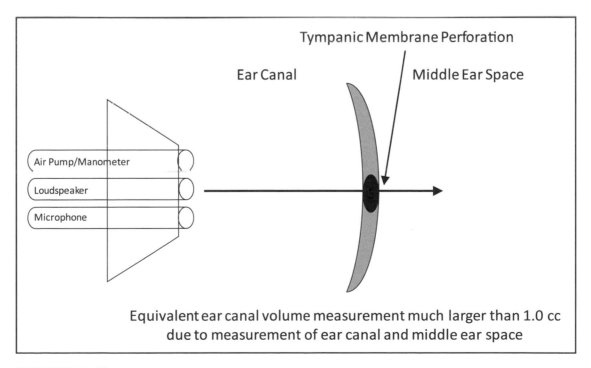

**FIGURE 5–17.** Measurement of large volume of air due to a tympanic membrane perforation.

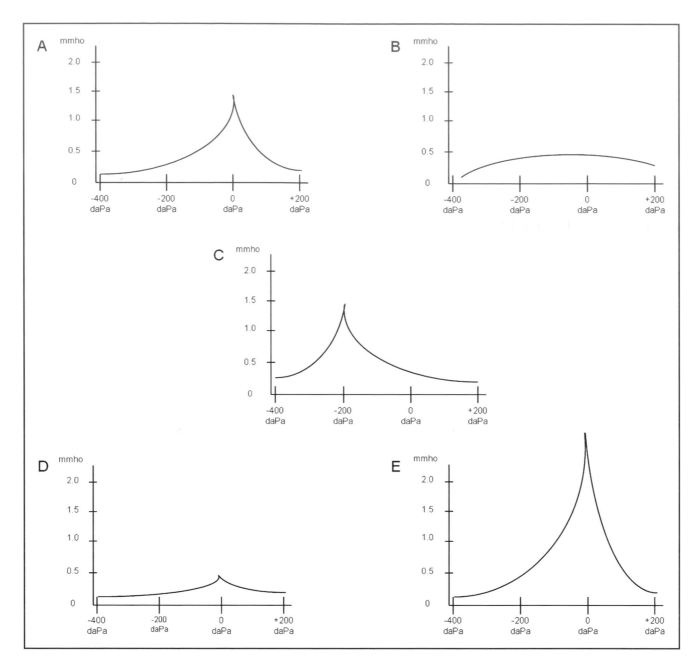

**FIGURE 5–18. A.** Type A tympanogram. **B.** Type B tympanogram. **C.** Type C tympanogram. **D.** Type A$_s$ tympanogram. **E.** Type A$_d$ tympanogram. Note that for conceptual understanding, the depth of the A$_d$ tympanogram is shown with the same scale as all other figures. Most immittance meters will rescale to provide a display of the entire tympanogram.

to expect. Specifically, it is helpful to instruct the patient that he or she will hear a tone and will feel some pressure in the ear. The probe for the unit must be situated in the ear so that an airtight seal is obtained and maintained throughout the test. If the seal is not present, the tympanogram will not run. Different size probe types are used for different sized ears. If a seal cannot be obtained with a given probe tip, it may be useful to select another size. When the probe is in place, the tympanogram should be started by pressing the appropriate button on the control panel of the equipment.

## OBSERVATION

1. Observe an experienced clinician prepare and provide instructions to a patient or volunteer for tympanometry.

2. Observe the clinician perform tympanometry on the patient or volunteer.

## GUIDED PRACTICE

1. Provide instructions to a patient or volunteer for tympanometry.

2. Obtain a seal in the ear canal using the probe from the immittance machine.

3. Obtain a tympanogram from a patient or volunteer.

4. Identify the static admittance, tympanometric peak, tympanometric width, and equivalent ear canal volume of the tympanogram.

5. Determine the type (shape) of the tympanogram.

6. Have another student perform tympanometry on you.

## REFLECTION AND REVIEW

1. After having tympanometry performed on your own ears, describe the sensations that you perceived during the test.

   _We felt a little burst of pressure followed by a peep, it was a weird sensation_

2. What is the frequency of the probe tone used for adults?

   _226 Hz_

3. What is the frequency of the probe tone used for children?

   _1000 Hz_

4. What happens if a patient or volunteer talks while the tympanogram is being recorded? Why does this occur?

_The seal could be broken causing an incomplete test._

5. What are the components of the immittance probe necessary for performing tympanometry?

_Air pump / manometer, loud speaker, microphone_

6. What are the units of measurement on the graph that make up the tympanogram?

_mmho_
_daPa_

7. What is the relationship between the amount of sound energy remaining in the ear canal and the admittance of sound energy into the middle ear space?

_♂ this could cause a flat result_

8. Describe what is meant by tympanometric static admittance.

_this is determined by the height of the peak_

9. Describe what is meant by tympanometric peak pressure.

_the pressure that occurs at the top of the peak_

10. Describe what is meant by tympanometric width.

_measure of width from ½ the static admittance to +200 daPa_

11. Describe what is meant by equivalent ear canal volume.

    measurment of volume of air infront
    of the probe

12. What type of pathology might you expect with a flat tympanogram and normal equivalent ear canal volume?

    tinitis media

13. What situations might cause an abnormally large equivalent ear canal volume?

    ossicular disarticulation normal TM,
    can see all of it, + allows measurement

14. Under what condition does optimal admittance of sound energy into the middle ear space occur?

    if there are no obstructions and if it
    has an air tight seal

15. What types of pathologies might you expect with a Type A$_d$ tympanogram?

    ⌐ stiffness of middle ear
    ↳ decrease in

16. What types of pathologies might you expect with a Type A$_s$ tympanogram?

    increase in middle ear stiffness

17. What is the advantage of performing tympanometry in conjunction with pure-tone audiometry?

    You can get a whole picture of
    what is working and what isn't
    working to determine a diagnosis

# ▌▌▌ 6 ▌▌▌

## Acoustic Reflex Thresholds

The acoustic reflex threshold measurement is a means of assessing the integrity of the acoustic reflex pathway. Dysfunction in this pathway can point to specific areas of pathology, especially when combined with tympanometry, pure-tone sensitivity, and speech audiometry data.

## LEARNING OUTCOMES

- Understand what the acoustic reflex is and how it is elicited.
- Understand the purpose of acoustic reflex threshold measurement.
- Be able to perform acoustic reflex threshold testing.
- Be able to interpret acoustic reflex threshold results.

## REVIEW OF CONCEPTS

### The Acoustic Reflex

The stapedius tendon is connected to the head of the stapes in the middle ear. The stapedius mus-

cle, from which the tendon emanates, is innervated by the stapedial branch of the facial nerve (cranial nerve VII). When the stapedius muscle contracts, the stapes footplate is displaced slightly in the oval window. This displacement causes a stiffening of the ossicular chain, which results in a decrease in admittance of sound energy from the ear canal to the middle ear space.

The acoustic reflex is a contraction of the stapedius muscle in response to loud sound. The contraction of the stapedius muscle occurs bilaterally. So, even when the stimulus is presented only to one ear, both stapedius muscles will contract. The reflex that occurs in the ear where the stimulus is presented is called the *ipsilateral reflex*. The reflex that occurs in the ear opposite to where the stimulus is presented is called the *contralateral reflex*.

### Terminology

In the earliest days of acoustic reflex threshold testing, technology had not yet been developed to record the reflex measurement in the same ear that the stimulus was presented (the ipsilateral reflex). Instead, the stimulus tone was presented to the test ear, while the reflex was recorded in the opposite ear. The primary use of this measure was as an assessment of retrocochlear function. The reflex was referred to as a left reflex when the stimulus was presented to the left ear and a right reflex when the stimulus was presented to the right ear. Later, the ability to elicit and measure the reflex in the same ear allowed for inference of middle ear function. To differentiate the pathways, the reflex that was elicited in the same ear in which the stimulus was presented became known as the ipsilateral reflex. The reflex that was elicited in the ear opposite that in which the reflex was elicited became known as the contralateral reflex. Because the stimulus elicits a reflex in both ears simultaneously, both the ipsilateral and contralateral reflexes occur due to stimulation of the test ear. When the right ear is stimulated and the reflex is recorded in the left ear, this is called a *right contralateral reflex*. When the right ear is stimulated and the reflex is recorded in the right ear, this is called a *right ipsilateral reflex*. When the left ear is stimulated and the reflex is recorded in the right ear, this is called a *left contralateral reflex*. When the left ear is stimulated and the reflex is recorded in the left ear, this is called a *left ipsilateral reflex*. A schematic demonstrating these relationships is shown in Figure 6–1.

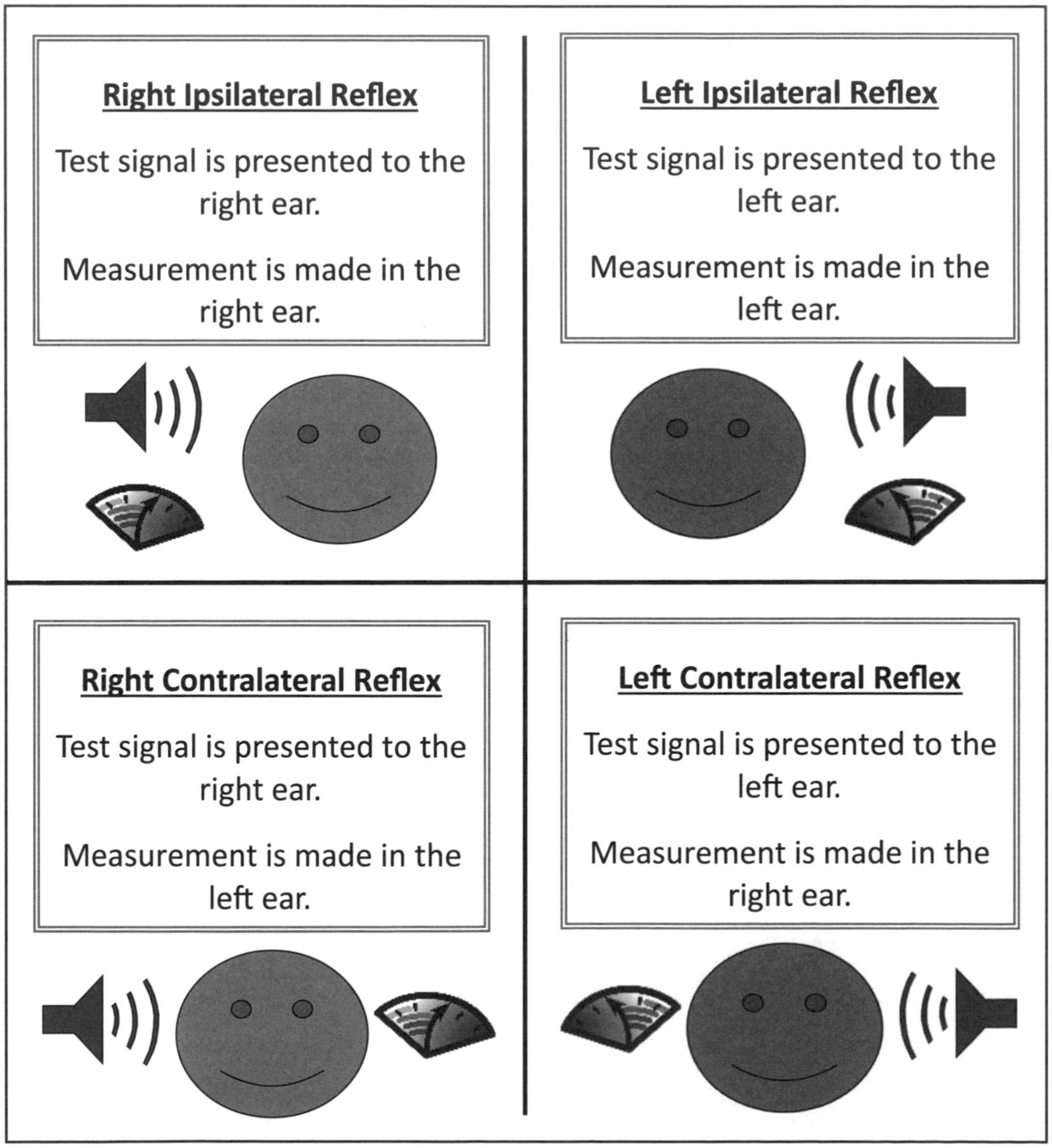

**FIGURE 6–1.** Terminology for acoustic reflexes.

## The Acoustic Reflex Pathway

Different neural pathways are involved in eliciting the ipsilateral and contralateral acoustic reflexes.

### *Ipsilateral Acoustic Reflex Pathway*

The ipsilateral acoustic reflex pathway includes the following components:

- ipsilateral middle ear
- ipsilateral cochlea
- ipsilateral VIIIth cranial nerve (acoustic) to the level of the ipsilateral ventral cochlear nucleus (VCN)
- ipsilateral VCN to the level of the superior olivary complex (SOC)
- ipsilateral SOC to the ipsilateral facial motor nucleus (FMN)
- ipsilateral VIIth cranial nerve (facial) to the stapedius muscle in the ipsilateral middle ear

A schematic of the ipsilateral acoustic reflex pathway is shown in Figure 6–2.

### *Contralateral Acoustic Reflex Pathway*

The contralateral acoustic reflex pathway includes the following components:

- ipsilateral (to the stimulus) middle ear
- ipsilateral cochlea
- ipsilateral VIIIth (acoustic) cranial nerve to the level of the ipsilateral ventral cochlear nucleus (VCN)
- crossover from the ipsilateral VCN to the contralateral superior olivary complex (SOC)
- contralateral SOC to the contralateral facial motor nucleus (FMN)
- contralateral VIIth (facial) cranial nerve to the stapedius muscle in the contralateral middle ear

A schematic of the contralateral acoustic reflex pathway is shown in Figure 6–3.

## Acoustic Reflex Threshold

The acoustic reflex threshold is the lowest intensity level at which the acoustic reflex is elicited with a particular stimulus. The stimulus levels are typically presented in 5 dB increments, just as they are for audiometric evaluation. Clinically, the acoustic reflex threshold typically is elicited both ipsilaterally and contralaterally to evaluate both acoustic reflex pathways. Frequencies typically tested include 1000 and 2000 Hz for ipsilateral reflexes and 500, 1000, and 2000 Hz for

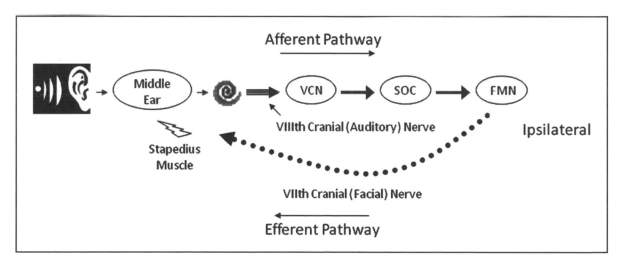

**FIGURE 6–2.** Ipsilateral acoustic reflex pathway. (FMN, facial motor nucleus; SOC, superior olivary complex; VCN, ventral cochlear nucleus.)

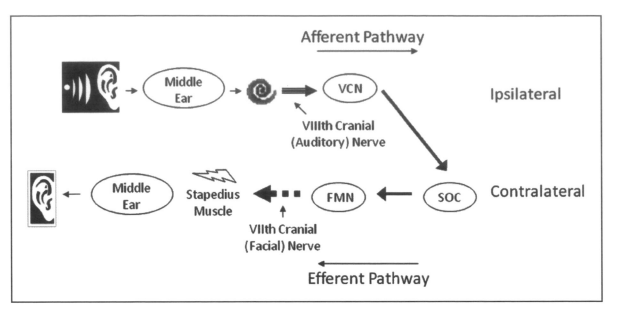

**FIGURE 6–3.** Contralateral acoustic reflex pathway. (FMN, facial motor nucleus; SOC, superior olivary complex; VCN, ventral cochlear nucleus.)

contralateral reflexes. Other stimuli, such as broadband noise, may be used as well.

## Performing Acoustic Reflex Threshold Testing

The same probe that is used to measure a tympanogram is used to determine the acoustic reflex threshold. In addition to having the components described earlier (i.e., air pump/manometer, microphone, and probe-tone loudspeaker), the probe unit contains another calibrated loudspeaker for delivery of the stimulus used to activate the ipsilateral acoustic reflex. A loudspeaker in the form of a probe or insert earphone is also placed into the contralateral ear for presentation of the contralateral stimulus. The measurement probe is placed into the ear in the same manner as for tympanometry, with an airtight seal being necessary.

The patient should be instructed to remain as still and quiet as possible. The patient should be informed that a series of loud sounds will be heard. The pressure utilized in acoustic reflex testing should be that of the tympanometric peak pressure, allowing for optimal transfer of sound energy into the middle ear space. A schematic of this transfer of energy is shown in Figure 6–4.

The probe-tone is used to elicit a baseline admittance level. When a stimulus of sufficient intensity is presented, the acoustic reflex response occurs. The contraction of the stapedius muscle causes a stiffening of the ossicular chain and a resulting change in the admittance of sound energy into the middle ear space. A schematic of this process is shown in Figure 6–5.

The change in the level of admittance over the time course of the occurrence of the stimulus presentation is graphically represented. The stimulus is presented at several different intensity levels for each stimulus frequency. The lowest intensity level at which a demonstrable change in admittance occurs is the acoustic reflex threshold. A schematic of a graphic representation of the acoustic reflex response is shown in Figure 6–6.

Average threshold level for the acoustic reflex is 85 dB SPL, with a normal range from 70 to 100 dB SPL. Reflexes are considered to be elevated when they exceed 100 dB SPL. Reflexes are considered to be absent when a reflex threshold cannot be elicited at the highest intensity level that can be generated by the equipment for the activator signal. This is generally around the level of 110 dB SPL.

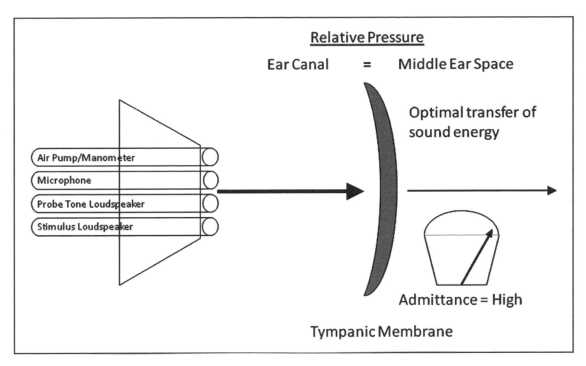

FIGURE 6–4. Process of measurement of probe-tone sound energy remaining in the ear canal.

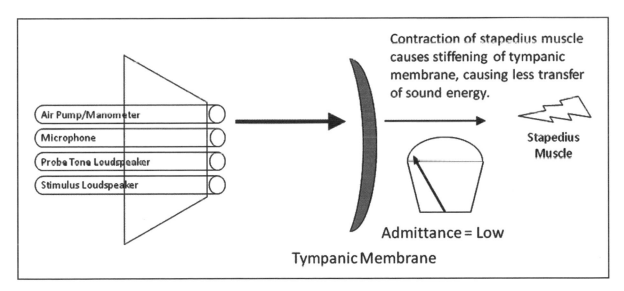

FIGURE 6–5. Stiffening of the tympanic membrane due to contraction of the stapedius muscle. The stiffness results in lower admittance of sound energy into the middle ear system and a greater degree of sound energy trapped in the ear canal.

## Normal Acoustic Reflex Patterns

An acoustic reflex pattern is considered normal when all four reflexes, right ipsilateral, right contralateral, left ipsilateral, and left contralateral, are present at normal threshold levels. This demonstrates the functional integrity of all components of both the ipsilateral and contralateral acoustic reflex pathways bilaterally. A representation of these normal findings is shown in Figure 6–7.

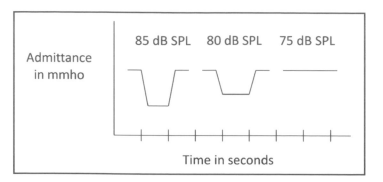

**FIGURE 6–6.** Graphic representation of the acoustic reflex response. Admittance of the probe-tone sound energy is plotted as a function of time. As the stimulus signal causes a contraction of the stapedius muscle, the tympanic membrane stiffens, resulting in a decrease in the admittance of sound energy into the middle ear space. This reduction is observed for the duration of the stimulus signal. Each stimulus signal plotted has a different intensity, which creates a different degree of contraction of the stapedius muscle. The lowest intensity, 75 dB SPL, results in no apparent contraction of the muscle. At 80 dB SPL, a demonstrable change in admittance is observed. The acoustic reflex threshold is 80 dB SPL.

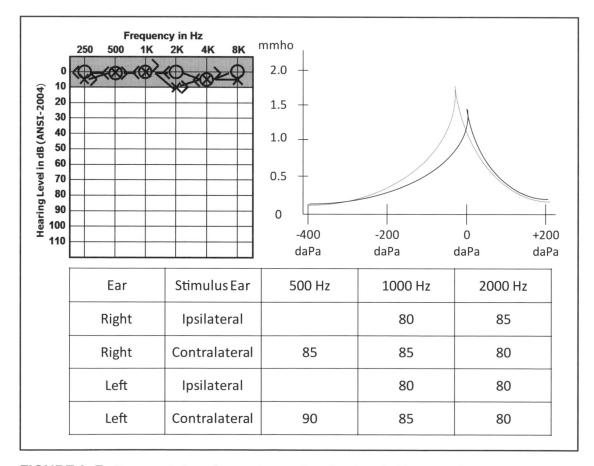

| Ear | Stimulus Ear | 500 Hz | 1000 Hz | 2000 Hz |
|---|---|---|---|---|
| Right | Ipsilateral | | 80 | 85 |
| Right | Contralateral | 85 | 85 | 80 |
| Left | Ipsilateral | | 80 | 80 |
| Left | Contralateral | 90 | 85 | 80 |

**FIGURE 6–7.** Representation of normal acoustic reflex thresholds, normal tympanometry, and normal hearing sensitivity.

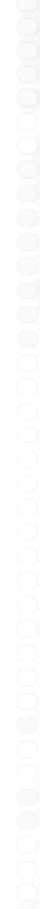

## Abnormal Acoustic Reflex Patterns

### *Unilateral Middle Ear Disorder*

In the case of unilateral middle ear disorder, an acoustic reflex will not be recorded from the probe in the disordered ear, due to abnormal function of the middle ear mechanism, a "probe effect." If there is a problem of admittance of sound energy into the middle ear space prior to the initiation of the stimulus tone, even if the stimulus could be made loud enough to cause a contraction of the stapedius muscle, no change reflective of the acoustic reflex can be recorded. A schematic demonstrating the location of breakdown in function in the acoustic reflex pathway due to unilateral middle ear disorder is shown in Figure 6–8.

Consider the following example. Imagine that the right ear has fluid in the middle ear space. The responses to right ipsilateral stimulation will be absent, because the response cannot be recorded due to middle ear dysfunction. The responses to left contralateral stimulation also will be absent because the response is being measured in the right ear and cannot be recorded due to middle ear dysfunction. The responses to right contralateral stimulation are elevated, because there is a conductive hearing loss in the right ear, which attenuates the intensity of the stimulus. The left

ipsilateral responses will be normal. Figure 6–9 shows an example of the pattern of acoustic reflex thresholds, tympanometry, and hearing test outcomes that could result from unilateral middle ear disorder.

### *Bilateral Middle Ear Disorder*

In the case of bilateral middle ear disorder, there is a "probe effect" bilaterally so that no responses are present in any configuration. A schematic demonstrating the location of breakdown in function in the acoustic reflex pathway due to bilateral middle ear disorder is shown in Figure 6–10.

Consider the following example. Imagine that both the right and left ears have fluid in the middle ear space. The stiffening effect of the fluid does not allow a change in stiffness to be recorded when, or if, the acoustic reflex is activated by the stimulus. Figure 6–11 shows an example of the pattern of acoustic reflex thresholds, tympanometry, and hearing test outcomes that could result from bilateral middle ear disorder.

### *Sensorineural Hearing Loss*

In the case of a sensorineural hearing loss, the resulting acoustic reflex responses will be dependent on the degree of hearing loss. For hearing

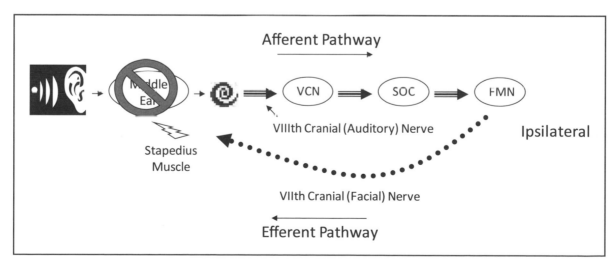

**FIGURE 6–8.** Location of breakdown in function in the acoustic reflex pathway due to unilateral middle ear disorder. (FMN, facial motor nucleus; SOC, superior olivary complex; VCN, ventral cochlear nucleus.)

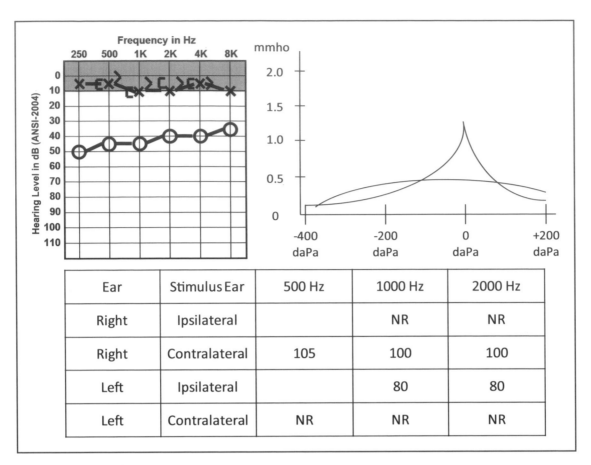

| Ear | Stimulus Ear | 500 Hz | 1000 Hz | 2000 Hz |
|---|---|---|---|---|
| Right | Ipsilateral | | NR | NR |
| Right | Contralateral | 105 | 100 | 100 |
| Left | Ipsilateral | | 80 | 80 |
| Left | Contralateral | NR | NR | NR |

**FIGURE 6–9.** Representation of acoustic reflex thresholds, tympanometry, and hearing test outcomes resulting from unilateral middle ear disorder.

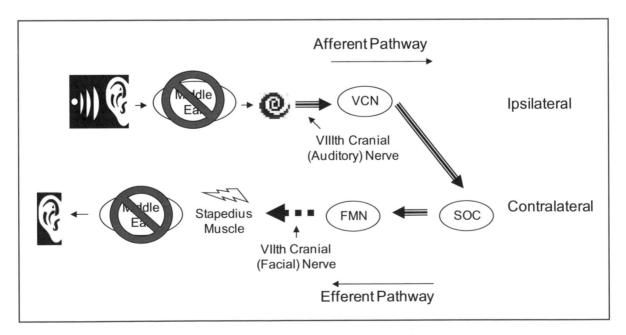

**FIGURE 6–10.** Location of breakdown in function in the acoustic reflex pathway due to bilateral middle ear disorder. (FMN, facial motor nucleus; SOC, superior olivary complex; VCN, ventral cochlear nucleus.)

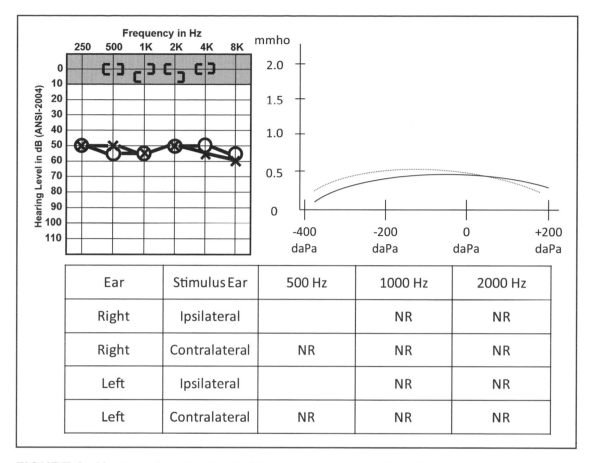

| Ear | Stimulus Ear | 500 Hz | 1000 Hz | 2000 Hz |
|-----|--------------|--------|---------|---------|
| Right | Ipsilateral | | NR | NR |
| Right | Contralateral | NR | NR | NR |
| Left | Ipsilateral | | NR | NR |
| Left | Contralateral | NR | NR | NR |

**FIGURE 6–11.** Acoustic reflex thresholds, tympanometry, and hearing test outcomes resulting from bilateral middle ear disorder.

losses less than about 50 dB HL, there generally will be no change in the acoustic reflex response. For thresholds between about 50 and 80 dB HL, acoustic reflex responses may be elevated. For thresholds greater than this, acoustic reflex responses will be absent. A schematic demonstrating the location of breakdown in function in the acoustic reflex pathway due to cochlear dysfunction is shown in Figure 6–12.

Consider the following example. Imagine that the right ear has a moderate sensorineural hearing loss and the left ear has a severe hearing loss, as shown in the audiogram. The effect of reduced sensation level affects the presence and level of the acoustic reflex response. Figure 6–13 shows an example of the pattern of acoustic reflex thresholds, tympanometry, and hearing test outcomes that could result from cochlear dysfunction.

### Retrocochlear Dysfunction

Dysfunction of the VIIIth cranial nerve (acoustic/vestibular), such as a vestibular schwannoma, can result in an absence of acoustic reflex responses when the stimulus is presented to the affected ear. A schematic demonstrating the location of breakdown in function in the acoustic reflex pathway due to retrocochlear dysfunction is shown in Figure 6–14.

Consider the following example. Imagine that the right ear has retrocochlear dysfunction due to a lesion of the VIIIth cranial nerve. Figure 6–15 shows an example of the pattern of acoustic reflex thresholds, tympanometry, and hearing test outcomes that could result from retrocochlear dysfunction.

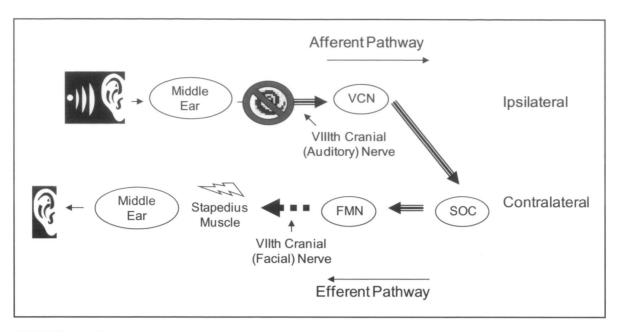

**FIGURE 6–12.** Location of breakdown in function in the acoustic reflex pathway due to cochlear dysfunction. (FMN, facial motor nucleus; SOC, superior olivary complex; VCN, ventral cochlear nucleus.)

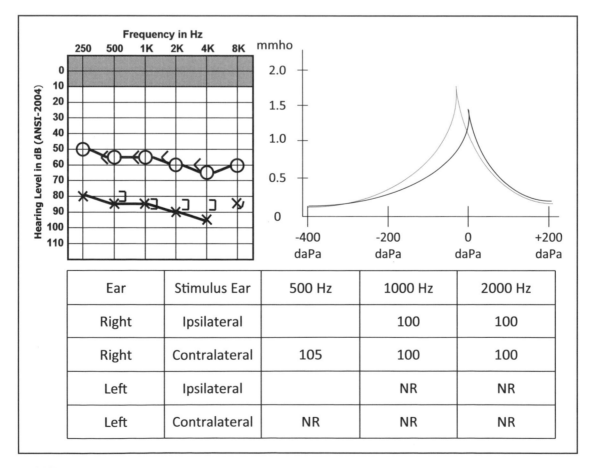

| Ear | Stimulus Ear | 500 Hz | 1000 Hz | 2000 Hz |
|---|---|---|---|---|
| Right | Ipsilateral | | 100 | 100 |
| Right | Contralateral | 105 | 100 | 100 |
| Left | Ipsilateral | | NR | NR |
| Left | Contralateral | NR | NR | NR |

**FIGURE 6–13.** Acoustic reflex thresholds, tympanometry, and hearing test outcomes resulting from cochlear dysfunction.

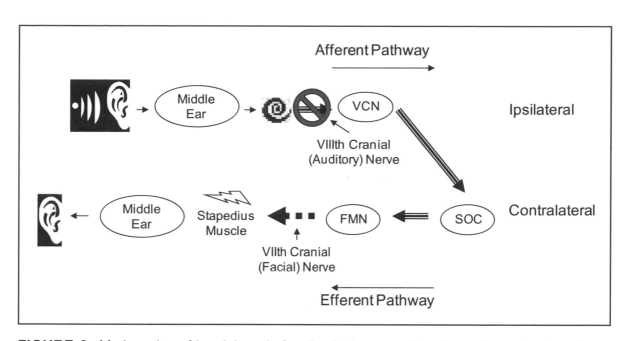

**FIGURE 6–14.** Location of breakdown in function in the acoustic reflex pathway due to retrocochlear dysfunction. (FMN, facial motor nucleus; SOC, superior olivary complex; VCN, ventral cochlear nucleus.)

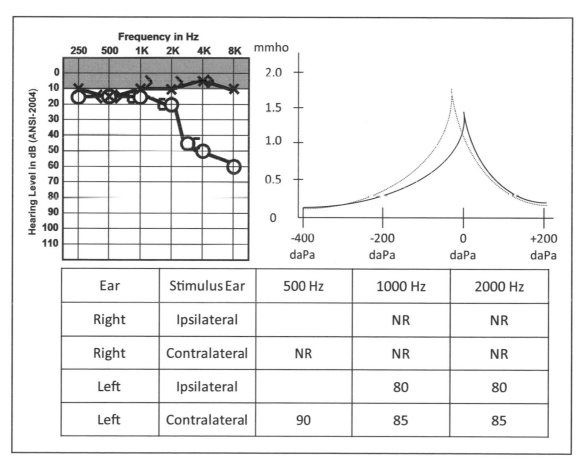

| Ear | Stimulus Ear | 500 Hz | 1000 Hz | 2000 Hz |
|---|---|---|---|---|
| Right | Ipsilateral | | NR | NR |
| Right | Contralateral | NR | NR | NR |
| Left | Ipsilateral | | 80 | 80 |
| Left | Contralateral | 90 | 85 | 85 |

**FIGURE 6–15.** Acoustic reflex thresholds, tympanometry, and hearing test outcomes resulting from retrocochlear dysfunction.

## Facial Nerve Dysfunction

Dysfunction of the VIIth cranial nerve (facial) results in the absence of an acoustic reflex response in the ear with the facial nerve damage, regardless of which ear is stimulated—a classic probe effect. A schematic demonstrating the location of breakdown in function in the acoustic reflex pathway due to facial nerve dysfunction is shown in Figure 6–16.

Consider the following example. Imagine that there is facial nerve dysfunction on the right side, with the left side being normal. There are no responses to right ipsilateral stimulation because the stapedius muscle on the right side does not contract. The responses with stimulation to the right side, recorded on the left side (right contralateral), are normal because this pathway is intact. There is an absence of response to stimulation of the left ear with contralateral recording (left contralateral) because the stapedius muscle on the right side does not contract, even with stimulation to the left ear. The left ipsilateral thresholds are normal. Figure 6–17 shows an example of the pattern of acoustic reflex thresholds, tympanometry, and hearing test outcomes that could result from facial nerve dysfunction.

## Third Window Effect

A reflex pattern may occur that demonstrates normal middle ear function in the presence of an apparent difference between air- and bone-conduction thresholds, known as an air-bone gap. The normal reflexes occur because there is normal function in reflex pathway. However, the air-bone gap may occur because of a phenomenon known as a third window effect where there is a pathologic area of mobility in the cochlear/semicircular canal structures. The result of a third window effect is that bone-conduction thresholds are artificially better when measured than they actually are (i.e., they are lower than they should be). This artificial lowering of the bone-conduction threshold creates an air-bone gap by decreasing the level of the measured bone-conduction threshold relative to the air-conduction threshold. In the case of a pure third-window effect, there is an artificial air-bone gap, but no conductive hearing loss and no middle ear dysfunction. This results in a pattern of an air-bone gap on audiometric testing, but a reflex pattern consistent with normal middle ear function. Figure 6–18 shows an example of the pattern of acoustic reflex thresholds, tympanometry, and hearing test outcomes that could result from a third window effect.

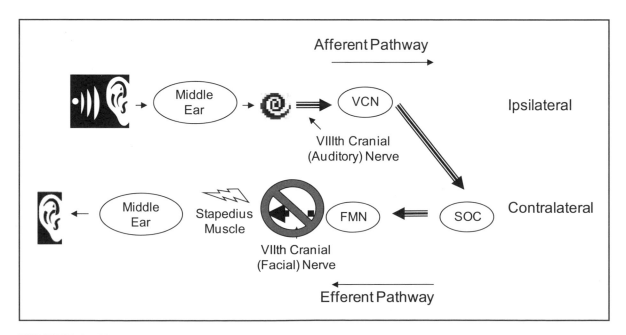

**FIGURE 6–16.** Location of breakdown in function in the acoustic reflex pathway due to facial nerve dysfunction. (FMN, facial motor nucleus; SOC, superior olivary complex; VCN, ventral cochlear nucleus.)

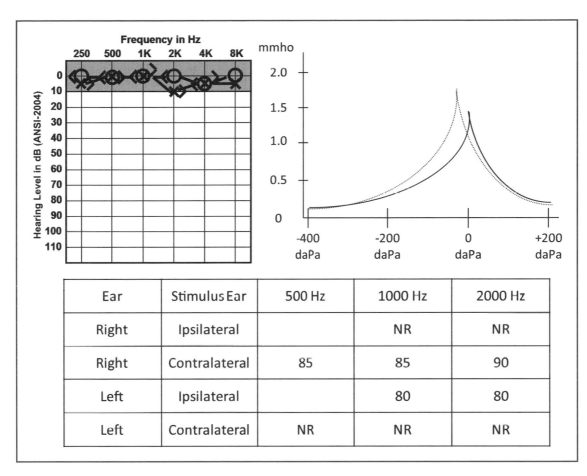

| Ear | Stimulus Ear | 500 Hz | 1000 Hz | 2000 Hz |
|-------|---------------|--------|---------|---------|
| Right | Ipsilateral | | NR | NR |
| Right | Contralateral | 85 | 85 | 90 |
| Left | Ipsilateral | | 80 | 80 |
| Left | Contralateral | NR | NR | NR |

**FIGURE 6–17.** Acoustic reflex thresholds, tympanometry, and hearing test outcomes resulting from facial nerve dysfunction.

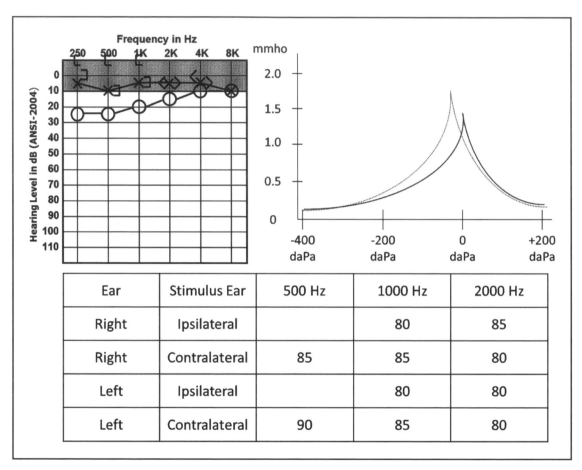

| Ear | Stimulus Ear | 500 Hz | 1000 Hz | 2000 Hz |
|------|-------------|--------|---------|---------|
| Right | Ipsilateral | | 80 | 85 |
| Right | Contralateral | 85 | 85 | 80 |
| Left | Ipsilateral | | 80 | 80 |
| Left | Contralateral | 90 | 85 | 80 |

**FIGURE 6–18.** Acoustic reflex thresholds, tympanometry, and hearing test outcomes resulting from a third window effect.

## OBSERVATION

1. Observe an experienced clinician instruct a patient or volunteer on what to do and what to expect during acoustic reflex threshold testing.

2. Observe the clinician obtain ipsilateral and contralateral acoustic reflex thresholds on a patient or volunteer.

## GUIDED PRACTICE

1. Prepare a patient or volunteer for acoustic reflex threshold testing by providing appropriate instructions and correctly placing the probe and contralateral earphone for testing of the right ear.

2. Obtain a tympanogram for the right ear.

3. Obtain ipsilateral acoustic reflexes for the right ear at 1000 and 2000 Hz.

4. Obtain contralateral acoustic reflexes for the left ear at 500, 1000, and 2000 Hz.

5. Reposition the probe and contralateral earphone for testing of the left ear.

6. Obtain a tympanogram for the left ear.

7. Obtain ipsilateral acoustic reflexes for the left ear at 1000 and 2000 Hz.

8. Obtain contralateral acoustic reflexes for the right ear at 500, 1000, and 2000 Hz.

9. Interpret responses to determine what the acoustic reflex thresholds reveal about the functionality of the acoustic reflex pathway.

## REFLECTION AND REVIEW

1. Describe the instructions you would provide to a patient on whom you are to perform acoustic reflex threshold testing.

   _____

   _____

   _____

   _____

   _____

2. Describe the process of obtaining an acoustic reflex threshold at a particular frequency.

   _____

   _____

   _____

   _____

   _____

3. Describe the entire process of obtaining a set of acoustic reflex thresholds.

   _____

   _____

   _____

   _____

   _____

   _____

4. What pattern of acoustic reflex thresholds would you expect when there is unilateral middle ear dysfunction?

_____

_____

_____

_____

5. What pattern of acoustic reflex thresholds would you expect when there is bilateral middle ear dysfunction?

_____

_____

_____

_____

6. What are some possible explanations for absent ipsilateral and contralateral acoustic reflexes bilaterally when there is severe hearing loss as measured by air conduction and other information is unknown?

_____

_____

# ||| 7 |||

## Acoustic Reflex Decay

### INTRODUCTION

Acoustic reflex decay is an objective measure used to assess retrocochlear function with immittance measurement methods. Abnormal decay can be a sign of retrocochlear dysfunction.

### LEARNING OUTCOMES

■ Understand the occurrence of acoustic reflex decay.
■ Be able to perform an acoustic reflex decay test.

### REVIEW OF CONCEPTS

The acoustic stapedial reflex occurs as a result of auditory stimulation. The reflex typically occurs for the duration of the stimulus. As the stimulus is presented continuously over time, however, the stapedius muscle contraction may diminish as the auditory system adapts to the stimulus. This phenomenon is known as *acoustic reflex decay*.

Acoustic reflex decay can be inferred using acoustic immittance measures similar to those used to observe acoustic reflex thresholds. In clinical situations, instead of the short-duration stimulus used in acoustic reflex threshold measures, a stimulus of about 10 seconds is presented. This stimulus is presented at 10 dB above the acoustic reflex threshold level to observe a robust acoustic reflex response. The stimuli used are 500 and 1000 Hz tones. Typically, the stimulus is presented to the ear contralateral to the ear with the probe. The resulting change in admittance of sound is observed at the onset of the stimulus, over the duration of the stimulus presentation, and at the stimulus offset. Under normal circumstances, the acoustic reflex decay will be less than half of the maximum change in admittance over the 10-second recording interval. A schematic of a normal acoustic reflex decay response is shown in Figure 7–1. In cases of abnormal acoustic reflex decay, the decay will be greater than half the maximum change in admittance during the course of the stimulus presentation. A schematic of an abnormal acoustic reflex decay response is shown in Figure 7–2.

Abnormal acoustic reflex decay raises suspicion of retrocochlear pathology that causes the auditory system to adapt too readily to acoustic stimulation. A tumor of the VIIIth cranial nerve is an example of a lesion that can cause abnormal

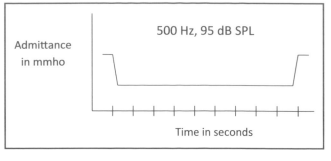

**FIGURE 7–1.** Normal acoustic reflex decay response.

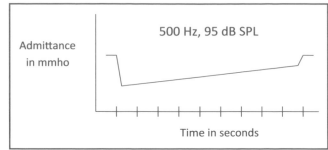

**FIGURE 7–2.** Abnormal acoustic reflex decay response.

acoustic reflex decay. In many cases of retrocochlear dysfunction, acoustic reflex thresholds will be absent at equipment limits or will be too high to present the stimulus tone. In these cases, acoustic reflex decay testing cannot be performed.

However, when acoustic reflex thresholds are at a level at which acoustic reflex decay testing can be performed at +10 dB SPL (re: the acoustic reflex threshold level), then this testing can be a useful addition to the diagnostic picture.

## OBSERVATION

1. Observe an experienced clinician perform acoustic reflex decay testing for a patient or volunteer.

## GUIDED PRACTICE

1. Write the instructions that you would give a patient prior to initiating the acoustic reflex decay test. Consider factors such as what the patient will perceive, whether the patient should remain still and quiet, and why you are completing the exam.

_____

_____

_____

_____

2. Prepare a patient or volunteer for acoustic reflex testing including insertion of probe and provision of instructions.

3. Obtain acoustic reflexes thresholds in the contralateral ear for 500 and 1000 Hz.

4. Perform acoustic reflex decay testing at 500 and 1000 Hz.

## REFLECTION AND REVIEW

1. Given acoustic reflex thresholds of 85 dB at 500 Hz and 90 dB at 1000 Hz, what should be the presentation levels of the stimuli for acoustic reflex decay testing at each frequency?

   _____

2. Examine the maximum output level for acoustic reflex decay for your immittance machine. What is the maximum threshold level of an acoustic reflex threshold that will still permit acoustic reflex decay testing?

   _____

3. How does acoustic reflex decay testing contribute to the comprehensive audiologic exam?

   _____

   _____

   _____

4. Will normal middle ear function be necessary to complete the acoustic reflex decay test? Why or why not?

   _____

   _____

   _____

# ||| 8 |||

## Audiometer Instrumentation

### INTRODUCTION

The audiometer is the essential tool of the audiologist for measuring hearing function. In this chapter, you will explore your audiometer and become familiar and comfortable with its use.

*Note:* Every style and model of audiometer is different. Some of the controls and options that are addressed in this chapter may not be available on the audiometer you are using. Nevertheless, it is important to understand these functions, as you may encounter them on equipment in the future. Alternatively, the audiometer that you are using may have features and functions that are not addressed in this chapter. The authors encourage you to become familiar with these features and functions as well. The User Manual for your particular equipment is a helpful tool for understanding the various components of your audiometer.

### LEARNING OUTCOMES

■ Know the fundamental components of the audiometer.

■ Know the ranges of the various parameters of the audiometer you are using.
■ Become comfortable with manipulation of controls on the audiometer.
■ Be able to manipulate controls to present desired stimuli.

### REVIEW OF CONCEPTS

#### What Is an Audiometer?

An audiometer is an electronic instrument designed for the presentation of calibrated auditory stimuli to transducers. The transducers deliver the auditory signal to the patient. The buttons and knobs on the control panel are used to select the type of auditory signal presented (tones, noise, speech); characteristics of the signal presented, including frequency (when applicable) and intensity; and the transducer through which the signal is routed. Other controls are available on most audiometers, but these are the basic controls.

There are a variety of audiometers available on the market. Some audiometers are designed for screening purposes and have minimal controls and features available. Typically these audiometers consist of one channel—meaning that they deliver only one signal at a time. Other audiometers are designed for clinical use and have a number of components. Often, these are two-channel audiometers. This means that two different and independent signals can be delivered to one or both ears at the same time. Audiometers may be stand-alone or computer based. The components of audiometers described here are meant to be representative of stand-alone modern audiometers that are widely used in university clinical settings.

## Display and Control Panels

The display panel of the stand-alone audiometer is the location where the stimulus parameters are indicated. The display may look quite different depending on the type of audiometer used. The control panel is the location where audiometer controls are located. The user manipulates these controls to select the various parameters of the desired stimulus. A schematic of the display and control panels of an audiometer is shown in Figure 8–1.

## Interrupter Controls

Interrupter switches are controls used to present a signal. When the button on the instrument is pressed, the switch is activated, and the signal is on for the duration of time that the button is depressed. The "continuously on" buttons allow the signal to be presented when the button is pressed once, and remains on until the button is pressed again to turn the signal off. Alternatively, the signal presented by using the "continuously on" button can also be interrupted by depressing the interrupter button. A schematic of the "continuously on" and interrupter buttons of an audiometer is presented in Figure 8–2.

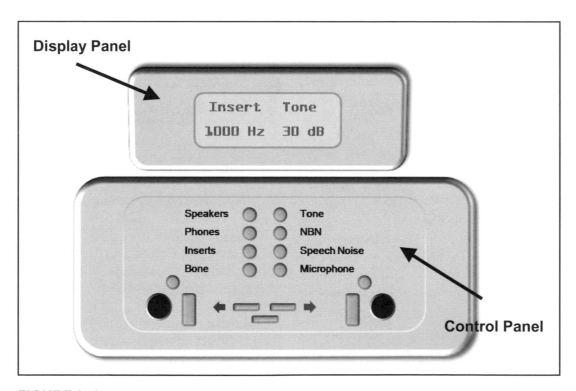

**FIGURE 8–1.** Display and control panels of an audiometer. The images shown in this chapter are modeled after the Grason-Stadler line of audiometers. (Permission courtesy of Grason-Stadler, Inc.)

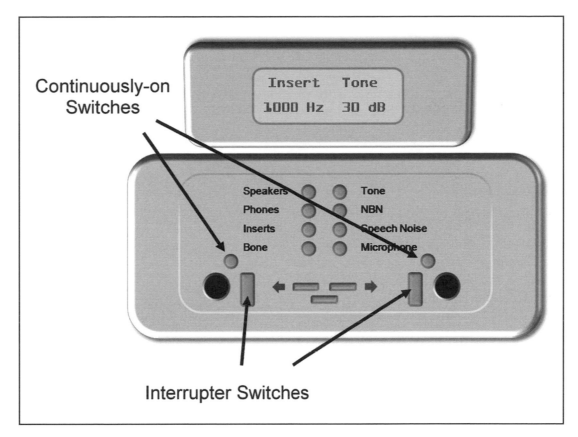

**FIGURE 8–2.** "Continuously on" and interrupter switches of an audiometer.

## Talk-Forward Switch and Monitor Control

A "talk-forward" switch is used to talk to the patient via a microphone for as long as the button is pressed. By pressing this button, the clinician is overriding any other settings on the audiometer momentarily. This signal is not calibrated. Inside the sound booth, there is a microphone, which transduces the auditory signal from within the sound booth, so that the examiner can hear what is being said in the testing room. The examiner may hear this via a headset with an earphone or via a loudspeaker housed within the audiometer. Most audiometers also have monitor controls, which allow the tester to listen to the stimuli as they are presented. A schematic of the talk-forward switch on an audiometer is shown in Figure 8–3.

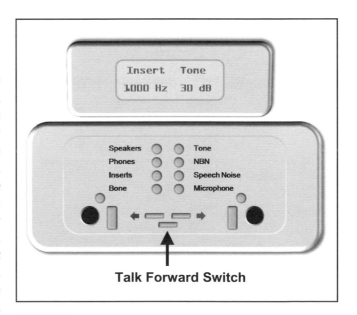

**FIGURE 8–3.** Talk-forward switch on an audiometer.

## Frequency Controls

The frequency control buttons are used to decrease or increase the frequency of the signal to be presented. Changes made using the frequency control buttons are shown in the display panel. A schematic of the frequency controls and frequency display are shown in Figure 8–4.

## Intensity Controls

Intensity controls are used to decrease or increase the intensity level of the signal to be presented. On most audiometers, changes made using the intensity controls are shown in the display panel and are completed by turning a dial. On others, intensity changes are made with push buttons. A schematic of the intensity controls and intensity display is shown in Figure 8–5.

## Signal Controls

There are buttons to control the type of signal presented. In some audiometers, changes made with the signal-type controls are shown in the display panel. Some signals are generated by the audiometer, such as pure tones and noise. Other signals are generated by external devices, such as a compact disc player, MP3 player, or computer input.

Live-voice also can be used as an input into the audiometer. When live-voice is used as the input, a volume unit (VU) meter allows the tester to visually monitor and adjust the level of the speech signal. A schematic of the signal controls and signal display is shown in Figure 8–6.

## Transducers

Several types of output transducers are used in audiometry: insert earphones, supra-aural earphones, loudspeakers, and bone vibrators.

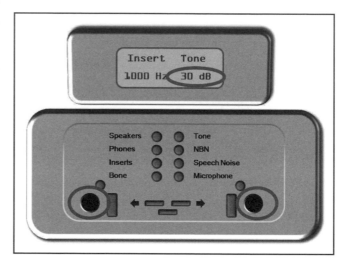

**FIGURE 8–5.** Intensity controls and intensity display.

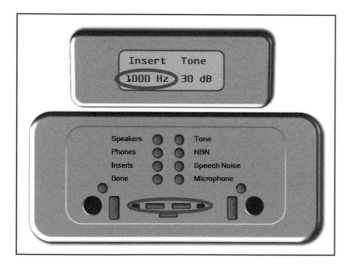

**FIGURE 8–4.** Frequency controls and frequency display.

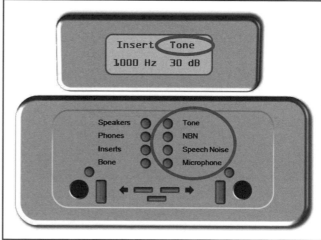

**FIGURE 8–6.** Signal controls and signal display.

Circumaural earphones may be used for high-frequency audiometry. Drawings of various transducer types are shown in Figure 8–7.

The type of transducer through which the audio signal is presented is controlled via switches on the audiometer. On some audiometers, changes made using the transducer controls are shown in the display panel. A schematic of the transducer selection controls and transducer type display is shown in Figure 8–8.

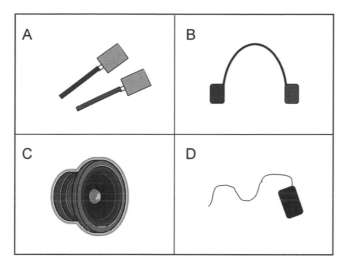

**FIGURE 8–7.** Various transducer types. **A.** Insert earphones. **B.** Supra-aural earphones. **C.** Loudspeakers. **D.** Bone-conduction transducer.

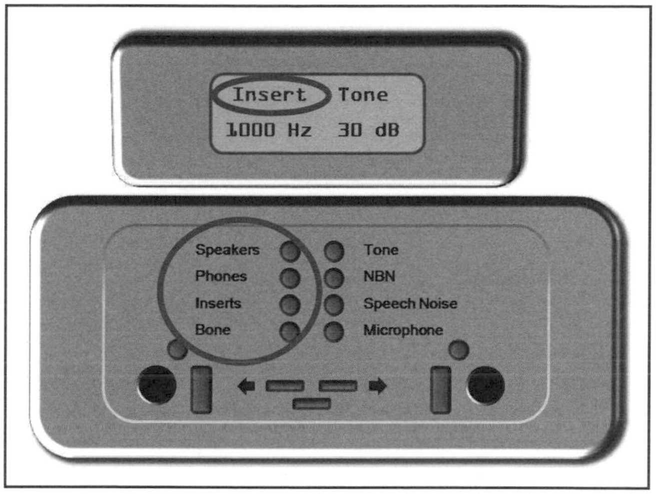

**FIGURE 8–8.** Transducer selection controls and transducer-type display.

## OBSERVATION

1. Observe an experienced audiologist completing an audiogram with a patient. Consider the speed with which the audiologist makes changes to the signal delivered to the patient.

2. Observe how the audiologist manipulates the controls of the audiometer to deliver desired signals to the patient.

## GUIDED PRACTICE

During this exercise, have a volunteer sit in the sound booth to listen to the sounds that you are generating. Also, have a volunteer perform these exercises while you listen in the sound booth.

*Note:* Be thoughtful and cautious about the signals that you are delivering to an individual's ears. High-intensity signals have the potential to permanently damage hearing. If the intensity of your presentation level continues to increase, but your volunteer does not perceive the signal, go back and verify your audiometer settings.

1. Find the power switch for the audiometer, and turn it on.

2. Look over the audiometer. Are you using a one-channel or two-channel audiometer?

_____

3. What is the make and model of the audiometer that you are using?

_____

4. When was the last date of calibration of the audiometer?

_____

5. Look at the back of the audiometer. Identify where the inputs into the audiometer are. Identify where the outputs from the audiometer are. What are the audiometer's inputs?

_____

6. What are the audiometer's outputs?

_____

7. Identify the controls for the audiometer. Determine where the controls are for transducer type, stimulus type, frequency, intensity, and interrupter switches.

8. Set the output to deliver tonal stimuli. Set the transducer to insert earphones. Change the frequency controls to determine the frequencies that the audiometer can deliver. What is the frequency range of the audiometer that you are using?

_____

9. Does the audiometer have a separate high-frequency control? If so, what is the high-frequency range of the audiometer?

_____

10. Keeping the output on tonal stimuli, change the intensity controls to determine the minimum and maximum output that the audiometer can generate. What is the intensity range for the audiometer at 1000 Hz?

_____

11. Change the frequency controls to determine how the intensity output varies with frequency. How does the intensity limit of the audiometer change for an 8000 Hz signal compared to a 1000 Hz signal?

_____

12. Change the transducer type to bone vibrator. How does the intensity limit of the audiometer change for a 250 Hz signal and a 4000 Hz signal? How does the maximum intensity output of the audiometer change for a bone vibrator compared to insert earphones?

_____

13. Set the transducer type to insert earphones. Set the output to tonal stimuli. Set the frequency level to 1000 Hz. Set the intensity level to 60 dB HL. Press the interrupter switch. Can you hear the tone at a comfortable level through the monitor speaker? If not, increase or decrease the monitor control to hear the tone at a comfortable level in the test booth.

14. Identify the microphone input to the audiometer. Set the signal type to microphone, and set the intensity level to 50 dB HL. Press the interrupter switch and talk into the microphone. Visualize the intensity of the input signal on the VU meter. Attempt to modify speaking so that speech peaks at the 0 level on the VU meter.

15. Determine whether there is a "continuously on" button. Use this button to deliver speech stimuli.

16. Look to see if the audiometer has a warble tone signal format. Present this type of tone to hear how it sounds. Present this type of tone using loudspeaker output.

17. Look to see if the audiometer has a pulsed tone signal format. Present this type of tone via earphones to hear how it sounds.

18. What are the noise-type options on the audiometer you are using?

_____

19. Listen to each type of noise to hear how it sounds.

20. Set the appropriate masking noise and frequency range to be on in one ear while the tonal stimulus is presented in the other ear. Verify that these stimuli are being presented correctly by asking your listener.

21. Set the audiometer to present an external input, such as from a CD player. Calibrate the signal using the calibration tone and the appropriate control on the audiometer by playing the "calibration tone" track and adjusting the input to 0 on the VU meter.

22. Present the external input at a comfortable listening level. Ensure that the listener can hear the stimuli. Observe the responses provided by the listener. Adjust talk-back volume as necessary to hear the listener's responses.

23. If possible, look at two different models of audiometers. Note similarities between the audiometers. How are the two audiometers you have examined different?

_____

_____

_____

## REFLECTION AND REVIEW

1. In what type of situations might it be necessary to use warble tones in a testing session? Why?

_____

_____

2. In what type of situations might it be useful to use pulsed tones in a testing session?

_____

3. What is the typical use of the noise stimuli?

_____

4. What other options are available on the audiometer that you are using that are not addressed here? What is the purpose of these functions?

_____

_____

_____

5. Why are the maximum outputs different for the transducers tested?

_____

_____

_____

6 Why is familiarity with the audiometer you are using critical in a clinical situation?

To be comfortable with your equiptment bc they are all different.

# III 9 III

## Biologic Check of Audiometer Instrumentation

### INTRODUCTION

Thorough electroacoustic calibration of audiometric equipment occurs on at least an annual basis. However, equipment malfunctions can happen at any time. It is difficult enough to discover that equipment is not working properly at the time that it is needed; it is even more distressing to discover that equipment has been working improperly but was undetected for an unknown period of time. Therefore, it is important to continually monitor the functionality of the equipment you are using. One easy method of doing this is to perform a daily biologic check of equipment. The term *biologic* is used to refer to a check of equipment by biologic means, in this case, listening to the equipment and determining its functionality by hearing. This is in contrast to an electroacoustic check of equipment, in which physical measurements are made to determine functionality of equipment.

### LEARNING OUTCOMES

■ Understand the purpose of performing a biologic check.
■ Know how to perform a biologic check for the audiometer.

### REVIEW OF CONCEPTS

To perform a biologic listening check, it is most efficient to have two people: one person to listen to the equipment and one person to control the equipment. The biologic check can be performed solo by using the "continuously on" button to present sounds while moving to the other side of the sound booth to listen.

A listening check should be performed with all transducers (insert earphones, supra-aural earphones, bone vibrator, and loudspeakers) to ensure that they are delivering signals appropriately. To check intensity, the level of the tone should be gradually increased to verify that loudness increases and is reasonably soft or loud depending on the level being presented. To check frequency, a tone should be presented while frequency is changed gradually. The listener should be able to perceive increases or decreases in pitch as this is manipulated. While performing this testing, cords should be moved about to determine that no static or other noises occur with movement. No other noises should be heard through the transducers when the signal is present. The signal should be perceived only in the selected transducer and not heard in any other transducers. If the signal is present in a transducer where it has not been routed, this is known as *cross-talk*.

The monitored live-voice and talk-back system should be activated with the listener talking to the presenter to determine whether this device is working. External inputs to the audiometer (such as compact disc players) should be checked and calibrated with the calibration tone.

In cases where there are problems with the equipment, the audiologist should troubleshoot equipment to determine whether there are obvious solutions for making equipment functional. Examples include equipment that is unplugged, jacks that are dirty and require cleaning, cords that are cracked or intermittent and need to be replaced, and external inputs that are not calibrated properly. When equipment has a problem that cannot be identified or cannot be fixed by the operator, the equipment should not be used until the problem can be repaired.

## GUIDED PRACTICE

1. Observe a clinician perform a biologic check of audiometric equipment.

2. Participate with a volunteer as a listener for a biologic check. Perform the following checks: visual inspection of equipment; listening check for intensity; listening check for frequency; and listening check for static, intermittency, and cross-talk.

3. Participate with a volunteer as a presenter for a biologic check.

4. Perform basic troubleshooting as necessary for equipment issues that are discovered.

## REFLECTION AND REVIEW

1. Describe the purpose of performing a daily biologic check.

_____

_____

_____

2. Describe the process of performing a daily biologic check.

   _____

   _____

   _____

   _____

   _____

3. Why is the biologic check important? What could be the worst-case scenario?

   _____

   _____

   _____

4. Develop a "checklist" for performance of a daily biologic check.

# Obtaining a Threshold

## INTRODUCTION

Obtaining an audiometric threshold is the most fundamental skill that you will learn as an audiologist. The ability to perform this task accurately and efficiently is an essential skill for audiologic practice.

## LEARNING OUTCOMES

- Understand the concept of threshold.
- Be able to obtain an audiometric threshold using the modified Hughson-Westlake method with a paper-and-pencil exercise.
- Be able to obtain an audiometric threshold using the modified Hughson-Westlake method with an audiometer and a volunteer listener.

## REVIEW OF CONCEPTS

### Threshold

An auditory sensitivity threshold is the softest sound that a person can hear. Figure 10–1 repre-

sents a theoretical "step-function" where, at given intensities, the patient would either not perceive the tone 100% of the time or would always perceive the tone 100% of the time. If patients actually perceived sound stimuli this way, determining threshold would be easy. Unfortunately, this is *not* how people perceive stimuli.

Figure 10–2 is a better representation of how people perceive stimuli. Many variables affect whether a person responds to a stimulus. At a

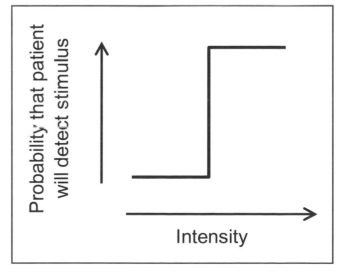

**FIGURE 10–1.** Step-function of perception demonstrating probability of detecting auditory stimuli as a function of intensity.

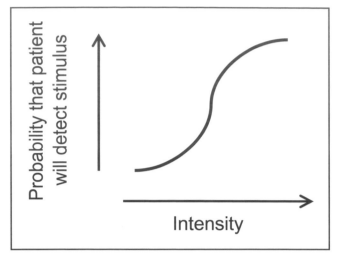

**FIGURE 10–2.** Continuous function of perception demonstrating probability of detecting auditory stimuli as a function of intensity.

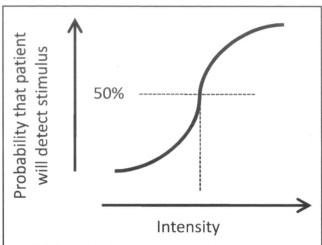

**FIGURE 10–3.** Continuous function of perception of auditory stimulus with 50% probability (threshold level) marked.

given intensity near threshold, sometimes they hear it, and sometimes they do not.

In clinical audiometric testing, we define the threshold of sensitivity as the lowest intensity level at which the patient responds 50% of the time. A demonstration of threshold on the function of perception is shown in Figure 10–3.

There are numerous ways to obtain a pure-tone threshold. We discuss the most commonly used procedure in audiology, called the *modified Hughson-Westlake procedure*.

## The Modified Hughson-Westlake Procedure

The modified Hughson-Westlake procedure is a "method of adjustment" for threshold determination. In the method of adjustment, a stimulus of a given intensity is presented. Depending on the patient's response (a positive response indicating that the sound was heard, or no response, indicating that the sound was not heard), the intensity level is changed, and another stimulus is presented.

With the modified Hughson-Westlake procedure, there are rules for determining what intensity to present depending on the patient's response. The rule is: "Down 10/Up 5." This

means that when a patient indicates that the sound has been heard, the next sound is presented at a 10 dB lower intensity. When a patient does not indicate that the sound is heard, the next sound is presented at a 5 dB higher intensity. This process continues until the patient responds to the tone at the same level at least 50% of the time on ascending (increasing intensity) runs.

Consider the following example. Suppose a patient is presented with a 30 dB HL tone at 1000 Hz as shown in Figure 10–4.

The patient responds to the tone. Following the "Down 10/Up 5" rule, the next tone is presented 10 dB lower, as shown in Figure 10–5.

Again, the patient responds to the tone. Following the "Down 10/Up 5" rule, the next tone is presented 10 dB lower, as shown in Figure 10–6. This time, the patient does not respond to the tone, so following the "Down 10/Up 5" rule, the next tone is presented 5 dB higher, as shown in Figure 10–7.

When the tone is presented the patient responds, so following the "Down 10/Up 5" rule, the next tone is presented 10 dB lower, as shown in Figure 10–8.

This time, the patient does not respond to the tone. Therefore, the next tone is presented 5 dB higher, as shown in Figure 10–9.

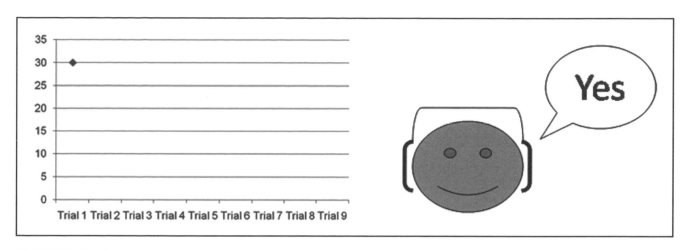

**FIGURE 10–4.** Trial 1: Affirmative patient response at 30 dB HL.

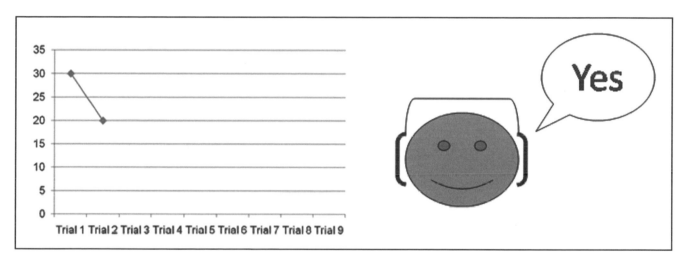

**FIGURE 10–5.** Trial 2: Affirmative patient response at 20 dB HL.

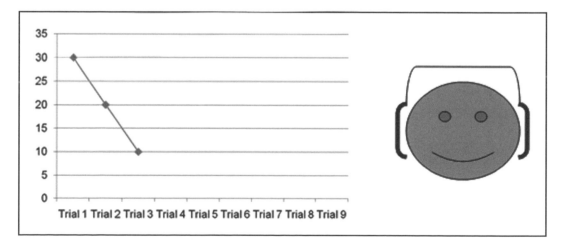

**FIGURE 10–6.** Trial 3: Negative patient response at 10 dB HL.

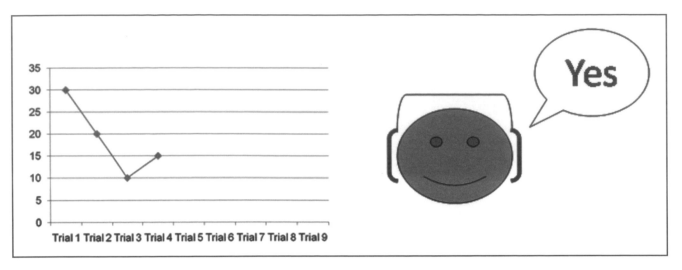

**FIGURE 10–7.** Trial 4:  Affirmative patient response at 15 dB HL.

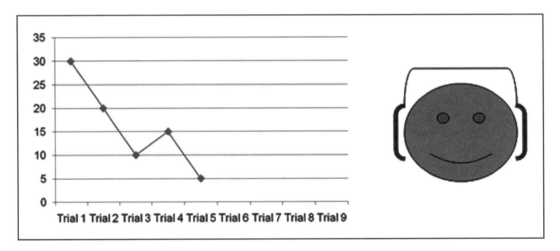

**FIGURE 10–8.** Trial 5:  Negative patient response at 5 dB HL.

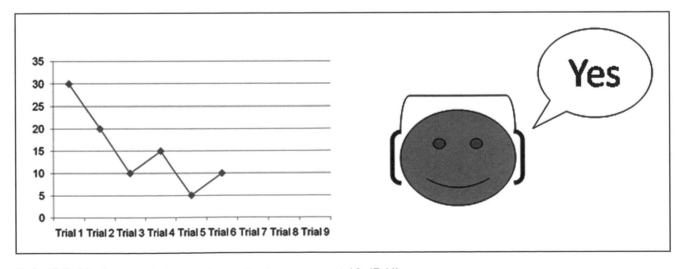

**FIGURE 10–9.** Trial 6:  Affirmative patient response at 10 dB HL.

When the tone is presented and the patient responds, the next tone is presented 10 dB lower, as shown in Figure 10–10.

The patient does not respond to this tone, so the next tone is presented 5 dB higher, as shown in Figure 10–11.

The patient again does not respond to the tone, so the next tone is presented 5 dB higher, as shown in Figure 10–12.

This time, the patient responds to the tone at 10 dB. This is the lowest level at which the patient responds to the tone on two ascending runs. Because this has occurred on two out of three runs, the criteria of the patient responding at least 50% of the time is fulfilled. This is the threshold.

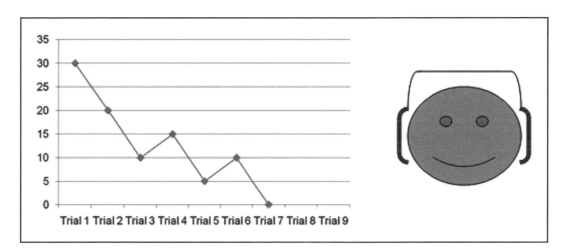

**FIGURE 10–10.** Trial 7: Negative patient response at 0 dB HL.

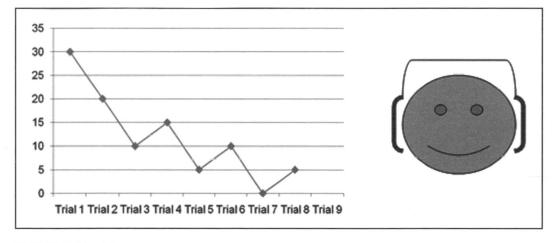

**FIGURE 10–11.** Trial 8: Negative patient response at 5 dB HL.

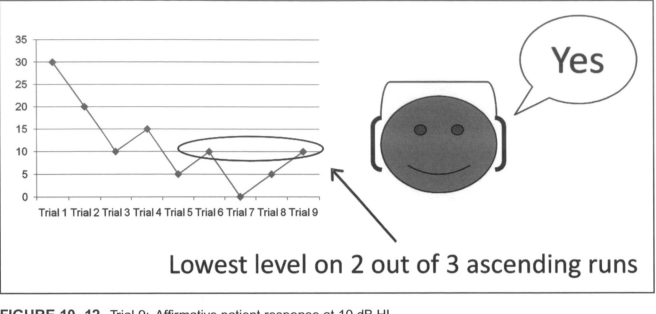

**FIGURE 10–12.** Trial 9: Affirmative patient response at 10 dB HL.

## OBSERVATION

1. Observe an experienced clinician obtain a pure-tone threshold on a patient or volunteer.

   a. What instructions does the clinician give to the patient?

   b. Why do you think that appropriate instructions are important for obtaining accurate thresholds?

   c. Does the clinician use a charting method to determine threshold, or is this process accomplished "in the head" of the clinician?

## GUIDED PRACTICE

1. Complete the following theoretical exercise to obtain threshold using the modified Hughson-Westlake procedure. Imagine that a volunteer is seated in the sound booth and you are about to find threshold in the right ear at 1000 Hz.

   a. What instructions do you give to the volunteer?

   _____

   _____

   _____

Use the graph presented in Figure 10–13 to chart your presentation levels and the volunteer's responses and your presentation levels to help you. *Note:* You may not need to use every trial on the chart for the task.

b. You present the first tone at 30 dB HL. The volunteer responds to the tone. According to the Down 10/Up 5 rule, what should you do?

_____

c. When you present the next tone, the volunteer responds to suggest that the tone was heard. The next tone should be presented at what intensity level?

_____

d. This time the volunteer does not respond to the tone. What do you do next?

_____

e. This time the volunteer does not respond to the tone. At what intensity level should you present the next tone?

_____

f. Once again, the volunteer does not respond to the tone. At what intensity level should you present the next tone?

_____

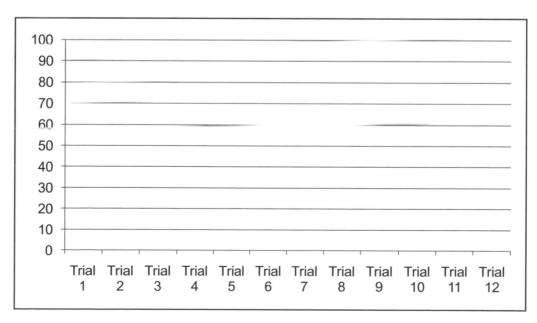

**FIGURE 10–13.** Graph for tracking patient response.

g. The volunteer responds to the tone at this level. What do you do next?

_____

h. This time, when you present the tone, the volunteer does not respond. At what intensity level should you present the next tone?

_____

i. At this level, the volunteer does not respond. At what intensity level should you present the next tone?

_____

j. The volunteer responds at this level. What do you do next? Have you found threshold? Why or why not?

_____

_____

2. Obtain threshold for a 1000 Hz tone on a volunteer under earphones using an audiometer. You can use the graph presented in Figure 10–14 to chart the patient's responses and your presentation levels to help you. Start at 30 dB HL and follow the modified Hughson-Westlake procedure (Down 10/Up 5) to obtain a threshold.

3. Have someone find your threshold at 1000 Hz.

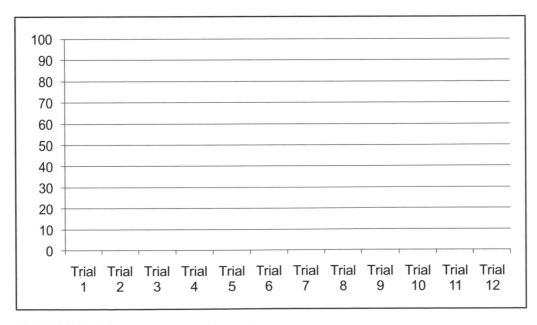

**FIGURE 10–14.** Graph for tracking patient response.

## REFLECTION AND REVIEW

1. Describe your experience with having your threshold obtained. Was it difficult to determine whether or not you heard the tone?

_____

_____

2. Imagine that you instructed the patient to be "absolutely sure" that he or she heard the tone; how might this impact your threshold results?

_____

_____

3. How do you think that you will recognize when patients are too willing to "guess" that they heard the tone?

_____

_____

4. How might the instructions that you give to a child be different from those that you give to an adult?

_____

_____

_____

_____

# ||| 11 |||

## Obtaining an Unmasked Air-Conduction Audiogram

## INTRODUCTION

Once you have learned about the concept of threshold and how to estimate an audiometric threshold, you will be able to expand that knowledge to obtain a measure of hearing sensitivity across frequencies, or an audiogram. In this chapter you will learn how to obtain an unmasked air-conduction audiogram.

## LEARNING OUTCOMES

■ Understand the audiogram and know the symbols most commonly used in audiometric testing.
■ Be able to instruct patients to obtain valid results.
■ Know the frequencies most commonly tested during pure-tone air-conduction testing.
■ Know when to test interoctave frequencies.
■ Be able to obtain an unmasked air-conduction audiogram.

## REVIEW OF CONCEPTS

### The Audiogram

An audiogram is a graph on which an individual's hearing thresholds are plotted in decibels hearing level (dB HL) as a function of frequency. An example of a typical audiogram is shown in Figure 11–1.

Intensity in dB HL comprises the $y$-axis. Unlike most graphs, the audiogram is "upside down" in that the lowest-intensity sounds are plotted at the top of the graph, and the highest-intensity sounds are plotted at the bottom. The typical audiogram has a range of −10 to 120 dB HL. Frequency comprises the $x$-axis. The typical frequencies displayed are between 125 and 8000 Hz.

The construction of an audiogram is specific. The American National Standards Institute (ANSI) has developed standards for how an audiogram should appear (ANSI, 2004). This makes it easy for someone looking at two different audiograms to see the same pattern of results. In order to understand the markings on the audiogram, a legend

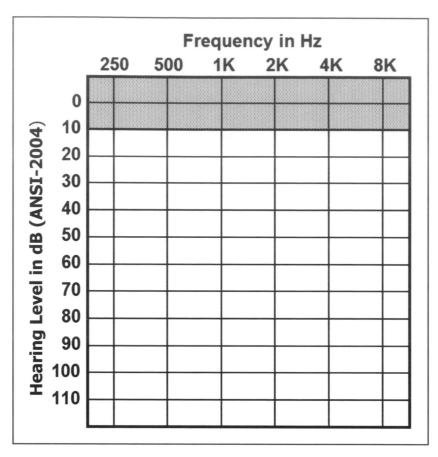

**FIGURE 11–1.** A typical audiogram.

typically is provided. A typical legend is shown in Figure 11–2. The symbols used in this manual are the same as those shown in Figure 11–2. For audiometric testing, there are different symbols to denote the specific ear tested (left or right), the type of transducer used (air-conduction or bone-conduction transducer), and whether or not masking was used in the other ear while the signal was presented (masked or unmasked). For example, to plot the unmasked air-conduction threshold for the left ear, an "X" symbol is used. This symbol is plotted on the graph at the intersection of the intensity determined to be threshold and the frequency that was tested. Imagine that the audiologist determined that the unmasked air-conduction threshold for the left ear was 30 dB HL at 1000 Hz. The threshold would be plotted as shown in Figure 11–3.

## Patient Preparation

Prior to beginning testing, the audiologist must physically prepare the patient and give instructions so that the patient will provide valid behavioral responses. The audiologist should ask the patient to remove food, chewing gum, glasses, and head coverings. If the patient is able to clearly see the tester from the other side of the booth, the patient should be seated so that the tester is not in direct view of the patient to avoid any visual cues that a signal is being presented.

To maximize patient comfort, the audiologist should explain each procedure and describe what will happen to the patient and what is expected of the patient at each step of the process. If other people are in the room with the patient, they should be instructed to be as quiet as possible

| Air Conduction | Bone Conduction |
|---|---|
| o right ear | < right ear |
| × left ear | > left ear |
| With Masking: | With Masking: |
| △ right ear | [ right ear |
| □ left ear | ] left ear |

| | | |
|---|---|---|
| * aided | S unaided | ↓ no response |

**FIGURE 11–2.** Figure legend for an audiogram.

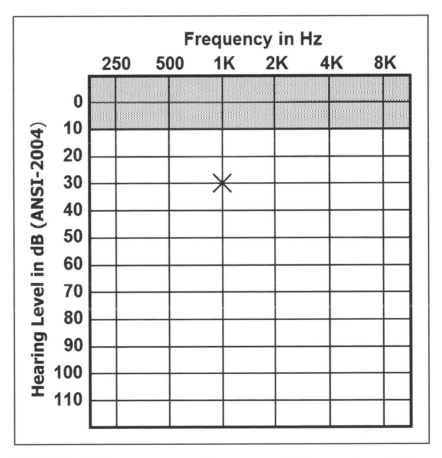

**FIGURE 11–3.** Audiogram with unmasked left ear air-conduction threshold of 30 dB HL at 1000 Hz.

to avoid interfering with the test. Typically, it is best for small children who are not being tested to wait outside the sound room and to minimize the number of people in the room. The patient also should be advised to minimize movement and any behaviors that produce sound.

Insert earphones should be the correct size for the patient's ear canal so that sound leakage does not occur. Insert earphones should be placed into the ear canal so that the foam tip is completely in the canal. The patient should be instructed prior to placement of earphones to maximize his or her potential to clearly hear and understand directions. When necessary, supra-aural earphones should be placed with transducer diaphragms covering each ear canal opening. Cords should be placed in back when possible so that patient does not have access to them.

The patient should be instructed to respond to the tone every time the tone is heard, as soon as it is heard. Patients should be told that the goal of the test is to find the softest level at which they hear. Therefore, the tones that they are listening for will be very soft, and they should respond when they hear the tone, even if it is very faint. The patient should be instructed as to how to respond, whether it is by pressing a response button, raising a hand, saying "Yes," or some other method. It often is helpful to instruct patients to respond in such a manner that the tester does not actually have to observe the patients in order to know that they have responded. This way, patients are not alerted to the presentation of the tone by the tester's associated observation of the patient.

You may find that some patients are more difficult to instruct than others. The concept of threshold is challenging for some listeners. For those who have difficulty understanding your directions, whether due to a language barrier, difficulty with communication due to hearing loss, cognitive limitations, dementia, or some other factor, instructions for the task will need to be made as simple as possible, and frequent reinstruction may be necessary.

## Testing Procedure

Begin with what the patient reports to be the better ear. If the patient does not report hearing better in one ear, begin with the right ear each time you test to avoid confusion.

Most clinicians test with continuous tone presentation. Use of pulsed tones can be advantageous when a patient has difficulty perceiving a continuous tone. For example, some patients with tinnitus report difficulty perceiving tones that are close in pitch to the presentation tone. Tones should be presented for about 1 s in duration.

The typical frequencies tested are 250, 500, 1000, 2000, 4000, and 8000 Hz. Interoctave frequencies should be tested whenever there is a difference of 20 dB or more between thresholds at adjacent octave frequencies. Some clinicians routinely test interoctave frequencies of 3000 and 6000 Hz as well.

Begin with 1000 Hz as this is a tone that is relatively easy to perceive. Find threshold using the modified Hughson-Westlake technique discussed in Chapter 10. Record the threshold on the audiogram using the appropriate symbol. Repeat this process for each frequency. Move on to testing 2000, 4000, and 8000 Hz. Retest 1000 Hz to ensure reliability of results. Then test 250 and 500 Hz.

## OBSERVATION

1. Observe an experienced clinician instruct a patient or volunteer how to respond to obtain valid pure-tone air-conduction results.

2. Observe a clinician obtain a pure-tone air-conduction audiogram.

## GUIDED PRACTICE

For Items 2 and 4 of the Guided Practice exercises, you may use the audiograms provided in Figures 11–4 and 11–5.

1. Physically prepare a patient for testing using insert earphones, and provide instructions to the patient.

2. Obtain an unmasked air-conduction audiogram for both ears using insert earphones.

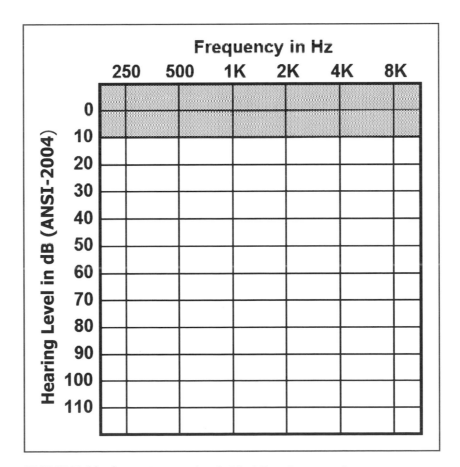

**FIGURE 11–4.** Audiogram for Guided Practice exercise.

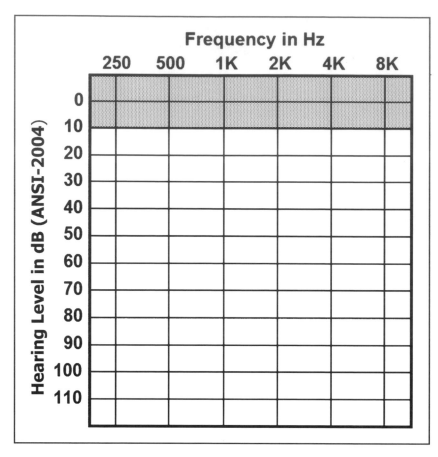

**FIGURE 11–5.** Audiogram for Guided Practice exercise.

3. Physically prepare a patient for testing using supra-aural earphones, and provide instructions to the patient.

4. Obtain an unmasked air-conduction audiogram for both ears using supra-aural earphones.

## REFLECTION AND REVIEW

1. Describe in detail the instructions you would provide to a patient on whom you are about to perform an unmasked air-conduction audiogram.

   _____

   _____

   _____

   _____

   _____

2. What frequencies are routinely tested for air-conduction audiograms?

   _____

3. When is it necessary to test interoctave frequencies?

   _____

4. Why is it useful to retest at 1000 Hz?

   _____

# ||| 12 |||

## Obtaining an Unmasked Bone-Conduction Audiogram

Once you have learned about the concept of threshold and how to estimate an audiometric threshold, you will be able to expand that knowledge to obtain any measure of hearing sensitivity. In this chapter, you will learn how to obtain an unmasked bone-conduction audiogram.

## LEARNING OUTCOMES

- Be able to describe proper placement of the bone vibrator.
- Be able to instruct patients to obtain valid results.
- Know the frequencies typically tested during pure-tone bone-conduction testing.
- Be able to obtain an unmasked bone-conduction audiogram.

## REVIEW OF CONCEPTS

### Patient Preparation

Prior to beginning testing, the audiologist must physically prepare the patient to be tested. A description of these methods can be found in Chapter 11. The bone vibrator should be placed with the appropriate side of the transducer on the mastoid bone of the patient. The headband should extend to the other side of the head, typically on the patient's temple. The bone vibrator should be positioned so that it is firmly against the mastoid and does not move easily. An alternative bone vibrator placement is on the forehead. In such a testing paradigm, a leather strap headband typically is used to hold the bone vibrator in place.

The patient should be instructed to respond to the tone every time it is heard, as soon as it is heard. Patients should be made aware that the tones are soft and that they should respond when they hear the tone, even if it is faint. Again,

95

reminding patients that the overall goal is to find the softest level at which they can hear typically is helpful. The patient should be instructed as to how to respond, whether it is by pressing a response button, raising a hand, saying "yes," or some other method. It is helpful to instruct the patient to respond in such a manner that the tester does not actually have to observe the patient to know that a response has occurred. This way, the patient is not alerted to the presentation of the tone by the tester's associated observation of the patient. When testing via bone conduction, it is helpful to instruct patients that they may hear the tone in either ear, and that they should respond every time they hear the tone, regardless of in which ear it is heard.

## Testing Procedure

For testing of unmasked threshold, begin with the bone vibrator on the mastoid of the ear with better air-conduction thresholds, or begin with the bone vibrator on the same ear each time if the thresholds between ears are symmetric. The typical frequencies tested for bone-conduction are 500, 1000, 2000, and 4000 Hz. Begin with 1000 Hz. Find threshold using the modified Hughson-Westlake technique discussed in Chapter 10. Move on to testing 2000, 4000, and 500 Hz. Some clinicians also test at 250 Hz, and may test at other frequencies as well, when knowledge of the bone-conduction threshold at additional frequencies is useful for differentiating between conductive and sensorineural hearing loss.

## OBSERVATION

1. Observe an experienced clinician instruct a patient or volunteer in how to respond to obtain valid pure-tone bone-conduction results.

2. Observe the clinician obtain a pure-tone bone-conduction audiogram using both right and left mastoid placement of the bone vibrator.

3. Observe the clinician obtain a pure-tone bone-conduction audiogram using forehead placement of the bone vibrator.

## GUIDED PRACTICE

For Items 2, 4, and 6 of the Guided Practice exercises, you may use the audiogram provided in Figure 12–1. All marks may be made on the same audiogram. Marks for forehead placement of the bone vibrator can be denoted on the audiogram with a "^" symbol.

1. Physically prepare a patient for testing using right mastoid placement of the bone vibrator, and provide instructions to the patient.

2. Obtain an unmasked bone-conduction audiogram with right mastoid placement of the bone vibrator.

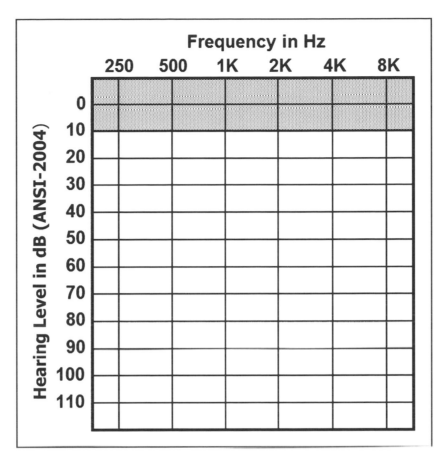

**FIGURE 12–1.** Audiogram for Guided Practice exercise.

3. Physically prepare a patient for testing using left mastoid placement of the bone vibrator, and provide instructions to the patient.

4. Obtain an unmasked bone-conduction audiogram with left mastoid placement of the bone vibrator.

5. Physically prepare a patient for testing using forehead placement of the bone vibrator, and provide instructions to the patient.

6. Obtain an unmasked bone-conduction audiogram with forehead placement of the bone vibrator.

## REFLECTION AND REVIEW

1. Describe in detail the instructions you would provide to a patient on whom you are about to perform an unmasked bone-conduction audiogram.

_____

_____

_____

_____

_____

_____

2. What frequencies are routinely tested for bone conduction?

_____

3. When testing for unmasked bone-conduction thresholds with the bone vibrator on the right mastoid, which ear is being stimulated? What about left mastoid placement? What about forehead placement?

_____

4. Why is it important to instruct the patient to respond to the tone, regardless of the ear in which it is heard?

_____

# ▎▎▎ 13 ▎▎▎

## Masking

Masking is one of the most challenging clinical concepts that audiology students encounter and one of the most difficult skills to master. However, the importance of masking cannot be overemphasized. When a stimulus is presented to one ear of a listener, there are occasions when the sound may be heard in the other ear due to bone conduction of the signal. The "fix" for this problem is to use noise in the opposite ear to mask the signal, so that the tester knows that the patient responses are due to hearing the signal in the ear being tested. Masking allows us to accurately evaluate the degree and type of hearing loss in each ear independently.

## LEARNING OUTCOMES

- Know what is meant by cross hearing.
- Be able to define interaural attenuation.
- Be able to define masking and describe its purpose.
- Know when to use masking.
- Know how to mask.
- Know about the "special issues" related to masking.

## REVIEW OF CONCEPTS

### Terminology

The following are some terms that will be used throughout the chapter:

The *test ear* (TE) (Figure 13–1) is the ear on which an audiogram is being determined.

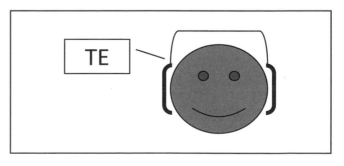

**FIGURE 13–1.** Test ear of the patient.

The *nontest ear* (NTE) (Figure 13–2) is the ear not being tested.

## Crossover

When testing hearing in the test ear, some sounds may be intense enough to stimulate the nontest ear. A schematic demonstrating this is shown in Figure 13–3. This is called crossover. Crossover happens by bone conduction. When the sound in the test ear is of sufficient intensity, it vibrates the bones of the skull, thereby stimulating the cochlea of the nontest ear. A schematic of how crossover occurs is shown in Figure 13–4.

## Cross Hearing

When the intensity of the sound that reaches the nontest ear exceeds the bone-conduction thresh-

old in that ear, the sound will be perceived. This is called cross hearing. A demonstration of this phenomenon is shown in Figure 13–5.

## What Is Masking?

Masking is the use of noise to prevent a test signal from being perceived in the nontest ear.

## Purpose of Masking

The goal of masking is to eliminate the ability of the nontest ear to "hear" the test signal by stimulating it with noise intense enough to disguise or "mask" the test signal in the nontest ear. An illustration of how the masking noise and test signals are presented is shown in Figure 13–6.

Masking ensures that, when a test signal is presented to the patient, the response of the patient is due to the test signal being perceived in the test ear instead of in the nontest ear. An illustration demonstrating this outcome is shown in Figure 13–7.

## Examples of Why Masking Is Necessary

The following examples demonstrate why masking is necessary in audiometric evaluation. Imagine

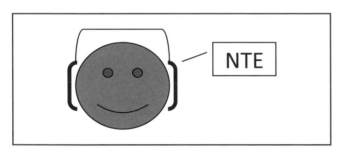

**FIGURE 13–2.** Nontest ear of the patient.

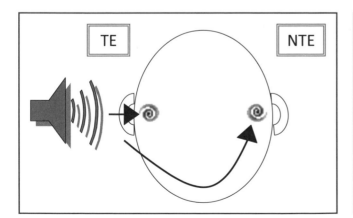

**FIGURE 13–3.** Crossover of acoustic stimulation to nontest ear.

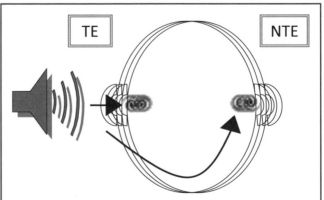

**FIGURE 13–4.** Crossover of acoustic stimulation to nontest ear occurs via bone conduction.

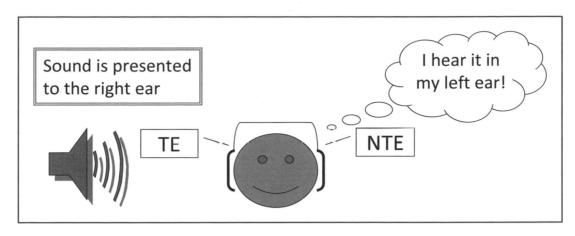

**FIGURE 13–5.** Demonstration of phenomenon of cross hearing.

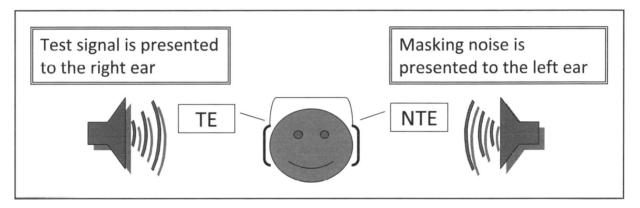

**FIGURE 13–6.** The masker is presented to the nontest ear to prevent it from hearing the stimulus presented to the test ear.

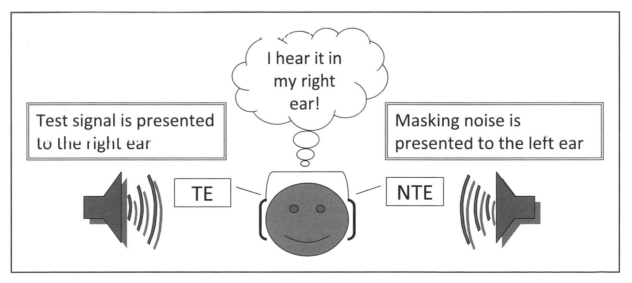

**FIGURE 13–7.** Appropriate behavioral outcome obtained by presenting masking noise to the nontest ear while presenting the stimulus to the test ear.

that a patient has normal hearing in the left ear and no hearing in the right ear (a "dead" ear). The audiogram accurately demonstrating this scenario is shown in Figure 13–8.

Figure 13–9 demonstrates what the audiogram might look like if masking is not used in the left ear while testing the right ear. Using insert earphones, the intensity of the signal presented by air conduction eventually will be great enough that the bones of the skull will vibrate, and the signal will be heard in the nontest (left) ear. Using the bone vibrator, the signal is heard in the nontest (left) ear at the same intensity level as if the stimulus were presented from the left mastoid because interaural attenuation can be as low as 0 dB for a bone-vibrator transducer. The resulting audiogram suggests that the patient has a severe conductive hearing loss in the right ear. This is not true. The presence of unmasked thresholds that

occur as a result of a sound being heard by crossover is known as a *shadow curve*. The appropriate use of masking noise in the left ear for air- and bone-conduction testing would provide the accurate results shown in Figure 13–8.

Another example of an unmasked audiogram is shown in Figure 13–10. In this case, the clinician must determine whether the hearing loss in the right ear is sensorineural, conductive, or mixed. To determine this, it is necessary to have accurate bone-conduction thresholds for the right ear. Without masking, the bone-conduction responses with the bone vibrator on the right mastoid are in the normal range. It may be that these thresholds are true and that the patient has a conductive hearing loss. Alternatively, it may be that the right bone-conduction thresholds are higher than these levels, reflecting a mixed or sensorineural hearing loss, but the bone-conducted signal is being

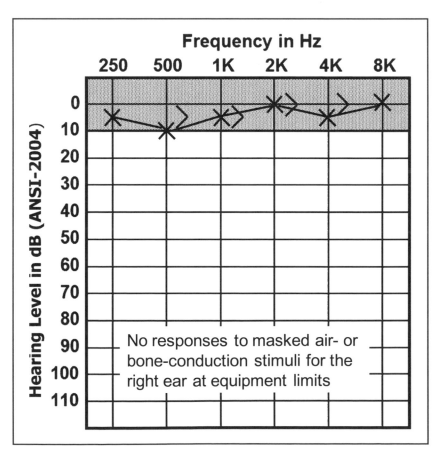

**FIGURE 13–8.** Audiogram of thresholds obtained for a "dead" right ear using masking in the left ear.

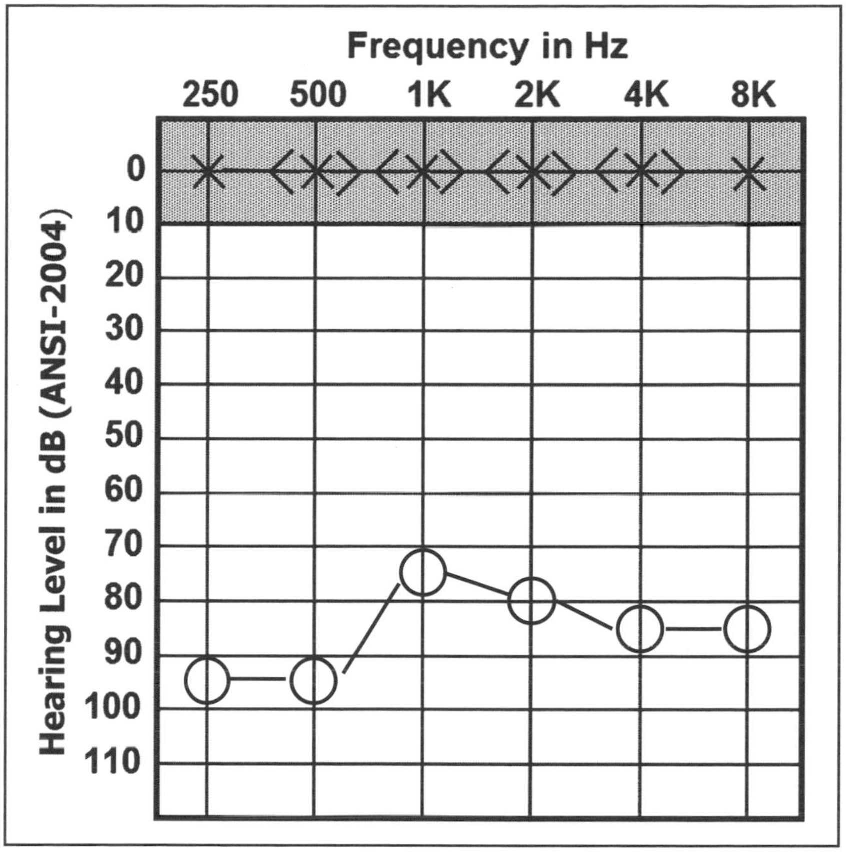

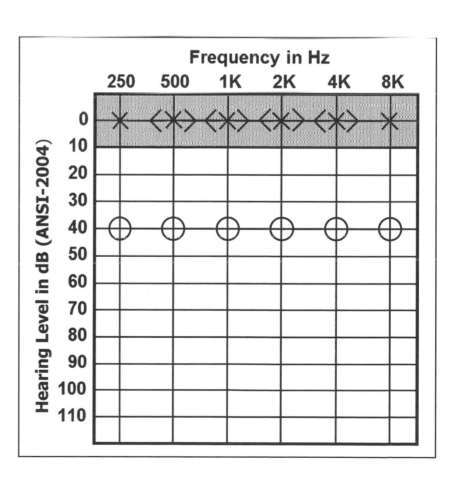

**FIGURE 13–9.** Audiogram showing results obtained for a "dead" right ear without masking the left ear.

**FIGURE 13–10.** Audiogram showing unmasked air- and bone-conduction thresholds.

perceived by the patient in the left ear, due to cross hearing. It is impossible to be certain of the validity of the right ear bone-conduction thresholds without masking the left ear.

Two different outcomes for this scenario are presented in Figures 13–11 and 13–12. In Figure 13–11, masking of the left ear allows the clinician to determine that the hearing loss is conductive. In Figure 13–12, masking of the left ear allows the clinician to determine that the hearing loss is sensorineural.

## How Does Masking Work?

A pure-tone signal is a signal of a particular frequency, such as a 1000 Hz tone of hypothetical amplitude, as shown in Figure 13–13.

A masking noise is a band of noise with a particular center frequency. In our example, the test signal is 1000 Hz, and the masking noise is composed of a narrow band of frequencies around 1000 Hz. The pure tone is shown in Figure 13–14A. The narrow band of masking noise is shown in Figure 13–14B.

The masking noise works to "cover up" the test signal. The test signal is still reaching the non-test ear due to crossover and still can be heard by cross hearing, but the masking noise does not allow the patient to perceive the test signal because it is embedded in the noise.

A visual example of masking is presented in Figure 13–15. The letter on the left side (Figure 13–15A) is not masked at all and can be clearly seen. The letter in the middle (Figure 13–15B) is somewhat masked visually but still can be seen.

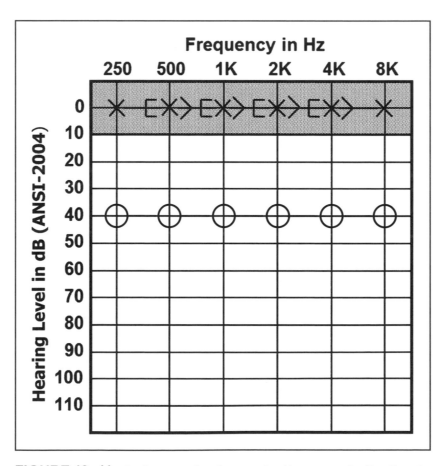

**FIGURE 13–11.** Audiogram showing masked bone-conduction thresholds for the right ear, indicating a conductive hearing loss.

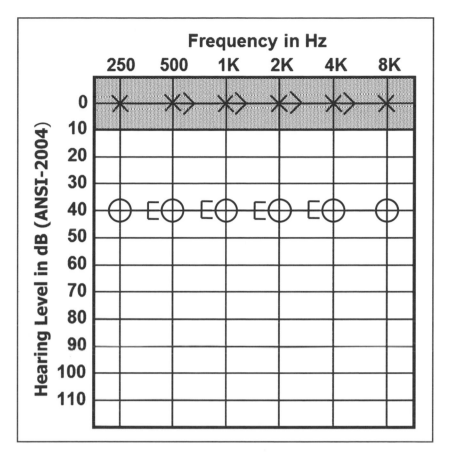

**FIGURE 13–12.** Audiogram showing masked bone-conduction thresholds for the right ear, indicating a sensorineural hearing loss.

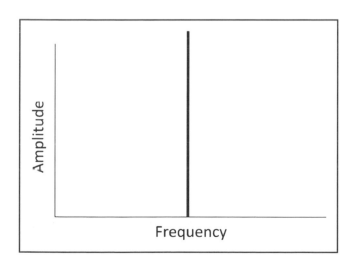

**FIGURE 13–13.** A 1000 Hz tone.

The letter on the right side (Figure 13–15C) is masked visually and can no longer be seen clearly. It is important to understand the letter is still there, but the reason that it cannot be seen is due to the masking. This concept of visual masking can be applied when considering auditory stimuli.

When using masking, crossover and cross hearing still are occurring, but the masking noise is covering up the test signal so that the patient does not respond to the test signal in the nontest ear. Because crossover and cross hearing are still occurring, the masking noise needs to be sufficient to mask the test signal.

### Interaural Attenuation

Crossover occurs by bone conduction. The test signal vibrates the bones of the skull, stimulating the cochlea of the nontest ear, as was shown in Figure 13–4. When the sound energy vibrates the bones of the skull, some sound energy is absorbed as the vibratory energy passes through the mass

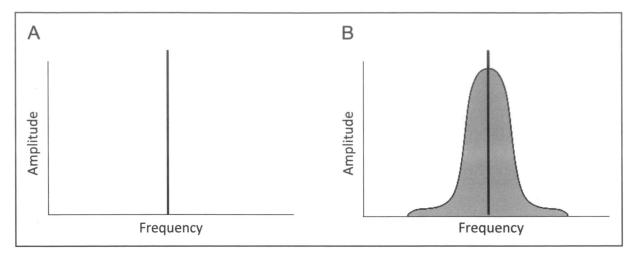

**FIGURE 13–14.** **A.** A 1000 Hz tone at a hypothetical amplitude. **B.** A 1000 Hz tone, masked by a 1000 Hz narrow band of noise. The band of noise "covers up" the pure tone with energy in the band of frequencies surrounding the pure tone.

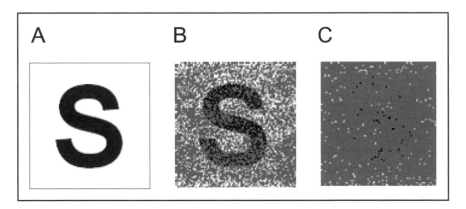

**FIGURE 13–15.** Visual example of masking. **A.** The letter is not masked at all and can be clearly seen. **B.** The letter is somewhat masked visually but can still be seen. **C.** The letter is masked visually and can no longer be seen clearly.

of the skull. The amount of sound energy lost as a result of this absorption is called *interaural attenuation* (IA). The amount of interaural attenuation for a given patient can be determined by subtracting the intensity of the signal reaching the nontest ear from the intensity of the test signal. The equation for this is

Intensity of test signal – intensity of signal reaching nontest ear = Interaural attenuation

Look at the example shown in Figure 13–16. An 80 dB HL signal is presented to the test ear. Twenty dB HL crosses over to the nontest ear. This means that 60 dB of sound energy was lost during crossover. The interaural attenuation is 60 dB.

Knowledge of the amount of interaural attenuation is necessary for determining whether the test signal is capable of stimulating the nontest ear. If the intensity level of test signal minus the interaural attenuation value is greater than or equal to

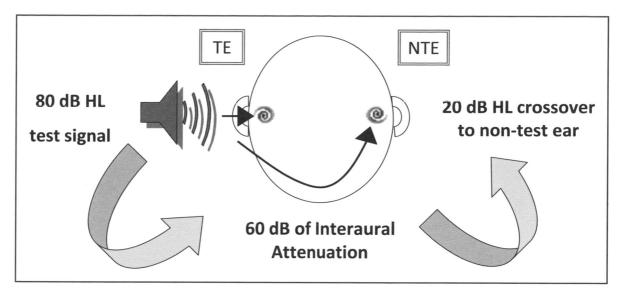

**FIGURE 13–16.** Example of calculation of interaural attenuation. An 80 dB HL test signal is presented to the test ear. Twenty dB HL crosses over to the nontest ear. Sixty dB of sound energy was lost during crossover. The interaural attenuation is 60 dB.

the bone-conduction threshold of the nontest ear, then the test signal is capable of being heard by crossover, and masking must be used.

Look at the example in Figure 13–16 again. An 80 dB HL signal is presented to the test ear. Twenty dB crosses over to the nontest ear. This means that 60 dB of sound energy was lost during crossover, and interaural attenuation is 60 dB. Now, consider what is happening in the nontest ear. It is known that 20 dB has crossed over to the nontest ear. But is the patient actually hearing the sound in the nontest ear? In other words, is cross hearing occurring? That depends on the patient's bone-conduction threshold for the nontest ear. Why the bone-conduction threshold? Because crossover happens by bone conduction. So, assume that the patient has a bone-conduction threshold of 30 dB HL in the nontest ear. Is the test signal being heard in the nontest ear? The answer is "No." Only 20 dB HL of sound intensity reached the nontest ear, and the patient requires at least 30 dB HL to hear the sound.

Assume now that the patient has a bone-conduction threshold of 10 dB HL in the nontest ear. Is the test signal being heard in the nontest ear? The answer is "Yes." There is 20 dB HL of sound

intensity reaching the nontest ear. This is more intense than the softest sound that the patient can hear. The patient perceives the sound and will respond.

To review, the interaural attenuation value is used to determine whether the sound will reach the other cochlea via crossover. If the sound reaches the nontest cochlea, then we must understand whether the sound may be heard by the nontest ear, which depends on the bone-conduction threshold of the nontest ear and how much the interaural attenuation has attenuated the intensity of the test signal. If the sound may be heard in the nontest ear, masking of the nontest ear is necessary.

Interaural attenuation values vary depending on several factors. The amount of interaural attenuation depends on the transducer that is used. Bone vibrators have the lowest interaural attenuation. Supra-aural earphones have intermediate values of interaural attenuation. Insert earphones have the highest interaural attenuation. This relationship is shown in Figure 13–17. So, a sound is most likely to be heard by crossover when using a bone vibrator. A sound is least likely to be heard by crossover when using insert earphones.

The amount of interaural attenuation also varies depending on the frequency of the test signal, as shown in Figure 13–18. In general, lower-frequency sounds have lower interaural attenuation, and higher-frequency sounds have higher interaural attenuation, although this relationship is somewhat different for insert earphones.

The amount of interaural attenuation also varies somewhat for each individual (Figure 13–19), so there is a range of values that occur as a result of individual differences.

When performing a hearing test, the actual interaural attenuation value for a given patient is unknown. To ensure that the nontest ear is not

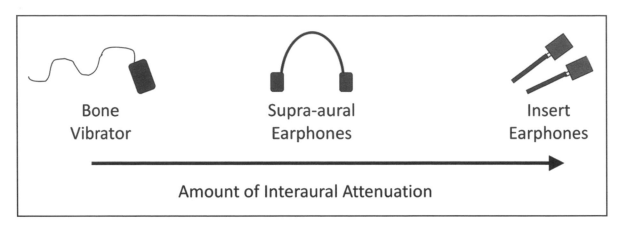

**FIGURE 13–17.** Relationship between the type of transducer and the relative interaural attenuation for each.

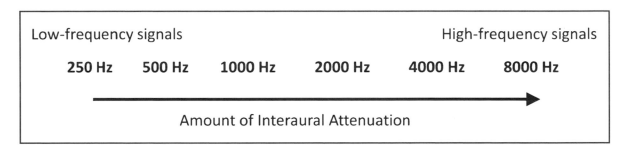

**FIGURE 13–18.** Relationship between frequency of test signal and relative interaural attenuation.

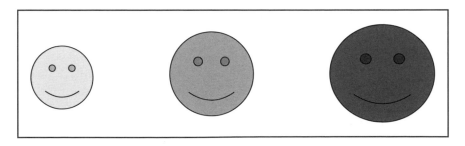

**FIGURE 13–19.** Hypothetical individual differences that contribute to differences in interaural attenuation.

accidentally tested, we use minimum interaural attenuation values. A minimum interaural attenuation value is the smallest interaural attenuation value for a given frequency and transducer type. These values have been determined empirically. Table 13–1 shows the minimum interaural attenuation values of the various types of transducers used in clinical audiometric testing.

Note how low the minimum interaural attenuation values are for the bone vibrator: 0 dB across the frequency range. Why is the minimum interaural attenuation value for the bone vibrator so low? It is because crossover and cross hearing happen via bone conduction. When the bone vibrator is directly causing vibration of the skull, it takes very little extra power to reach either cochlea.

As stated before, if the intensity level of the test signal minus the interaural attenuation value is greater than or equal to the bone-conduction threshold of the nontest ear, then the test signal is capable of being heard by crossover, and masking must be used. However, during clinical testing, we do not know what the actual interaural attenuation value is for a patient. So, we use the minimum interaural attenuation values to determine when masking is needed. The rule then becomes as follows: When the difference between the test signal and the bone-conduction threshold for the nontest ear is greater than or equal to the minimum interaural attenuation value for the test signal and the transducer used, then we must

**Table 13–1.** Minimum Interaural Attenuation Values (in dB) for Transducer Type and Frequency

| Transducer Type | Frequency (Hz) | | | |
|---|---|---|---|---|
| | 250 | 500 | 1000 | 2000 |
| Bone vibrator | 0 | 0 | 0 | 0 |
| Supra-aural earphones | 40 | 40 | 40 | 45 |
| Insert earphones | 95 | 85 | 70 | 75 |

*Sources:* Katz, J., & Lezynski, J. (2002). Clinical Masking. In J. Katz (Ed.), *Handbook of Clinical Audiology.* (pp. 124–141). Philadelphia, PA: Lippincott Williams & Wilkins; Killion, M. C., Wilber, L. A., & Gudmundsen, G. I. (1985). Insert earphones for more interaural attenuation. *Hearing Instruments, 36,* 34–36.

assume that there is a possibility that the test signal could be heard by crossover in the nontest ear, and masking must be used.

## How to Mask

### Audiometer Controls

Stimuli are presented via one channel of the audiometer, and masking noise is presented via the other channel. The intensity of the masking noise can be raised or lowered independently of the test ear signal using the attenuator dial. The type of masking noise is dependent on the type of signal being presented to the patient. Narrowband noise signals are used for masking of tonal stimuli. On most audiometers, the frequency band of the narrowband noise changes automatically to match the frequency of the tone selected for presentation. Speech-shaped noise is used to mask speech stimuli.

The intensity level of masking noise stimuli are calibrated to an effective masking level (EML). This level has been predetermined to be a sound pressure level (SPL) that effectively masks a signal of a given intensity in decibel effective masking level (dB EML). For example, a 30 dB EML narrowband noise centered at 1000 Hz effectively masks a 30 dB HL pure tone at 1000 Hz.

When determining threshold using masking noise, the masking noise is introduced using the "continuously on" control. This allows the masking noise to be presented continuously, while the test stimuli are presented intermittently. If the masking noise was presented only with the test stimuli, the patient would be alerted to the presentation. Therefore, the masking noise must be presented continuously to the nontest ear while threshold is established in the test ear.

### Patient Instructions

The instructions that are provided to the patient for masking are vital to obtaining valid responses from the patient. For many patients, simply providing responses to pure-tone stimuli alone can be a challenging task. Masking adds an auditory signal that the patient must ignore, while responding to test stimuli, which complicates the task further.

Here are some example instructions: "Now you are going to hear those same tones again. This time you will hear some 'wind' noise in your other ear. Just ignore the wind noise, but continue to say 'yes' every time you hear the tones." It is then helpful to present the masking noise to the patient and to reiterate that this is the type of sound that should be ignored. In some cases, patients will provide a false-positive response when the masking noise is introduced. It is necessary to reinstruct the patient when this occurs.

## Undermasking

When a masking signal is presented to the nontest ear, the intensity of the masking noise must be great enough that it covers up the signal crossing over from the test ear and being heard in the nontest ear. If it does not, then "undermasking" occurs. Recall the visual example in Figure 13–15. In image "B," the letter is undermasked and can still be seen.

## Overmasking

When a masking signal is presented to the nontest ear that is of a high intensity, it may be so high that the masking noise actually crosses over to the test ear by bone conduction. If it is intense enough, this can cause the test ear to also be masked. When you are testing, this would result in the observed threshold increasing every time the masking noise is increased. This is known as overmasking.

## Effective Masking

In between undermasking and overmasking is a level known as effective masking. This level of masking occurs when the masking noise is of a high enough intensity to effectively cover up the signal crossing over from the test ear but is low enough that the masking noise is not being heard by crossover in the test ear. Figure 13–20 illustrates this concept graphically.

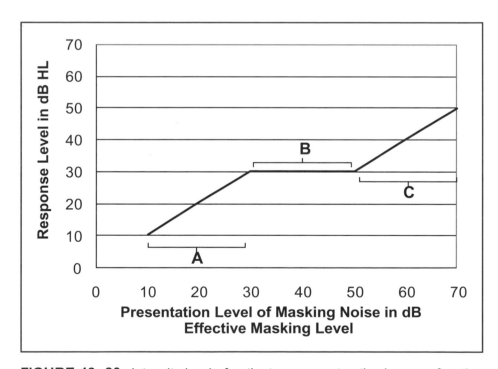

**FIGURE 13–20.** Intensity level of patient response to stimulus as a function of masking intensity. In section *A*, the masking noise and patient responses increase together in a linear function. This is the area of undermasking. In section *B*, increases in masking noise to do not cause changes in the level of the patient response. This is the "plateau" level and demonstrates an effective level of masking noise. In section *C*, the masking noise and patient responses again increase together in a linear function. This is the area of overmasking.

The portion of the function at the lower masking intensities shows that masking noise and patient responses increase together in a linear manner (Area A). This is the area of undermasking. Every time the intensity of the masking noise increases, the intensity level at which the patient responds increases. At the initial masking level, there is not enough intensity to sufficiently mask the signal that is being presented to the patient's test ear. This signal is crossing over to the nontest ear, is being heard by the patient, and the patient is responding. Each time the masking noise is increased in intensity, it takes a little more intensity of the test signal to reach the nontest ear, so the patient responds at the higher intensity level. This function continues until it reaches an area known as the "plateau."

The plateau of the function (Area B) represents a range where there is no change in the intensity level at which the patient responds, despite increases in the intensity level of the masking noise. At this point in the masking process, the intensity level of the masking noise is high enough to cover up the stimulus being presented to the test ear. We know this because, if it were not, the patient's response level would continue increasing with increases in the masker level. The intensity level of the masking noise is also not too intense. We know this because, if it were too intense, the patient's response level would again continue to increase with increases in the masker level as the masking noise is heard by crossover in the test ear. This plateau level is the "just right" area for masking. When the patient has at least three instances of providing responses at the same level despite increases in the masking noise intensity, you can safely consider the response level to be the patient's threshold in the test ear.

Area C on the graph represents the area of overmasking. Overmasking occurs when the masking noise presented to the nontest ear is crossing over to the test ear and is so intense that it causes the masking noise to be heard in the test ear. This causes the signal presentation to the test ear to be masked as well, and causes the patient response to be raised in that ear. The level at which the patient responds continues to rise with every increase in masking noise intensity. This pattern of responses creates a linear function where the patient's response level increases with each increase in masking noise.

### Plateau Method

The observation of the plateau of the patient's response function has led to the concept of the "plateau method" as a useful technique for clinical masking. In the plateau method, the audiologist first obtains an unmasked threshold. Then, the audiologist presents masking noise to the nontest ear at a level just above (10 dB greater than) the patient's air-conduction threshold for the nontest ear.

*Clinical Note:* There is an exception to the rule for how much masking noise to present initially. Generally the intensity should be 10 dB above the air-conduction threshold for the nontest ear. However, for the lower frequencies 250, 500, and 1000 Hz, more masking noise may be initially introduced. This is because of a phenomenon known as the *occlusion effect*. Correcting for the occlusion effect when presenting the initial intensity level essentially is a "shortcut." In order to not confuse the reader who is new to the plateau method, the occlusion effect shortcut will be ignored for now. We return to it later in the chapter.

With the initial masking level presented to the nontest ear, the threshold is reestablished in the test ear. The intensity of the masking noise is then raised by 5 dB, and the threshold of the test ear is again reestablished. As the intensity of the masking noise increases, the observed threshold level in the test ear will either increase in intensity or stay the same. When the threshold is increasing with consecutive increases in intensity of the masking noise, either the intensity level of the masking noise is insufficient to mask the test signal (undermasking), or the intensity level of the masking noise is being heard by crossover in the test ear and effectively raising the threshold (overmasking). When the threshold level has remained the same over three consecutive intensity increases, then the plateau of the function has been reached, and it can be safely determined that an effective level of masking noise has been used to obtain the masked threshold in the test ear.

Due to test/retest variability, it may be possible to obtain a reestablished threshold that does not shift when it should, or shifts when it should not. This is part of the reason why obtaining the same threshold at several masking intensity levels (the plateau of the function) is useful, as it allows us to observe the trend of the patient's response to the masking noise.

Here is an example. Assume that you have obtained unmasked air-conduction thresholds for the left ear and for the right ear using insert earphones and unmasked bone-conduction thresholds. You have obtained the audiogram shown in Figure 13–21. Note that the right air-conduction responses have the potential to have been heard by crossover in the left ear. This is because the minimal interaural attenuation for insert earphones (see values in Table 13–1) is greater than the bone-conduction thresholds for the left ear. This means that the stimuli used to obtain the unmasked right air-conduction thresholds could

have been heard by crossover in the left ear, causing the patient to respond. To determine whether the air-conduction thresholds are accurate, masking noise must be presented to the left ear.

You will use the plateau method to mask for air-conduction for the right ear. Begin at 1000 Hz. Narrow-band noise will be presented to the left ear to cover up the signal being heard in the left ear. At what intensity level should the noise be presented? The air-conduction threshold in the left ear is 0 dB HL. Using the plateau method, add 10 dB EML of masking noise to the nontest ear air-conduction threshold. Why are we worried about the air-conduction threshold when cross hearing occurs due to bone conduction? It is because masking noise is presented via air conduction. So, begin by presenting 10 dB EML of masking noise to the left ear. After reestablishing threshold, it is found that the air-conduction threshold

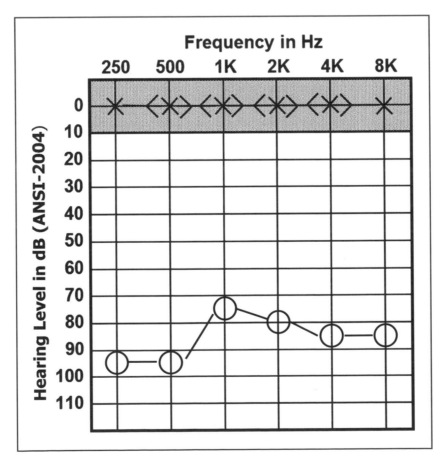

**FIGURE 13–21.** Audiogram showing unmasked air- and bone-conduction thresholds for the left and right ears.

has shifted to 85 dB HL as shown in the graph in Figure 13–22.

Following the plateau method, you then add another 5 dB EML to the masking noise. You reestablish the air-conduction threshold in the right ear and find that it shifts another 5 dB as shown in Figure 13–23.

Yet again, following the plateau method, you add another 5 dB EML to the masking noise. You reestablish the air-conduction threshold in the

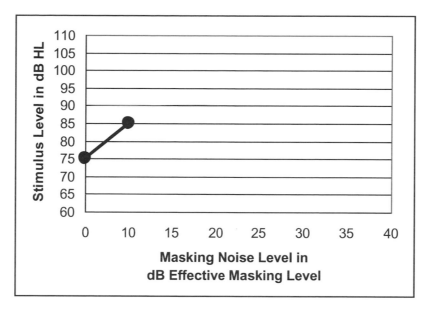

**FIGURE 13–22.** Patient response level as a function of presentation level of masking noise. There is a shift in threshold with addition of masking noise.

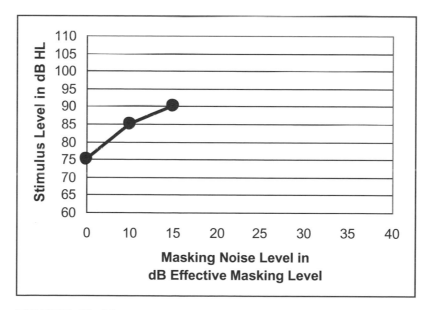

**FIGURE 13–23.** Patient response level as a function of presentation level of masking noise. There is an additional shift in threshold with higher masking noise intensity. The additional threshold shift suggests that this is an area of undermasking.

right ear and find that it shifts another 5 dB as shown in Figure 13–24.

This same procedure is followed again with the same results as shown in Figure 13–25.

Once again, you raise the masking noise by 5 dB EML and reestablish the air-conduction threshold in the right ear. This time, the threshold does not shift. It remains at 100 dB HL as shown in Figure 13–26.

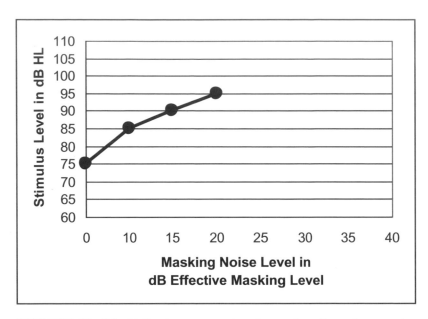

**FIGURE 13–24.** Patient response level as a function of presentation level of masking noise. There is an additional shift in threshold with higher masking noise intensity. The additional threshold shift suggests that this is an area of undermasking.

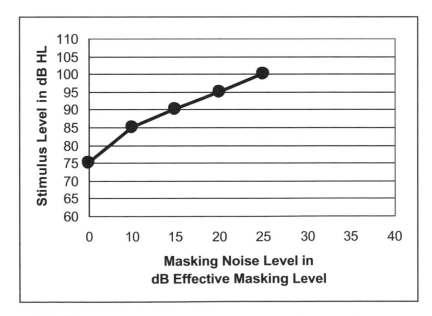

**FIGURE 13–25.** Patient response level as a function of presentation level of masking noise. There is an additional shift in threshold with higher masking noise intensity. The additional threshold shift suggests that this is an area of undermasking.

Following the plateau method, you repeat the process of raising the masking noise level by 5 dB EML. Again, you find that the threshold does not shift, as shown in Figure 13–27.

Once you have obtained at least three levels at the plateau, it is generally safe for you to stop masking. Just to be thorough, you once again repeat the process of raising the masking noise level by 5 dB EML. Again, you find that the threshold does not shift, as shown in Figure 13–28.

The masked air-conduction threshold has been determined to be 100 dB HL. Assuming a sensori-

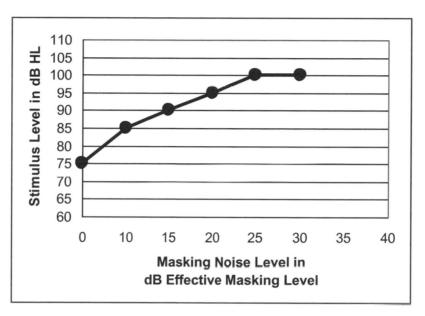

**FIGURE 13–26.** Patient response level as a function of presentation level of masking noise. There is no change in threshold with higher masking noise intensity.

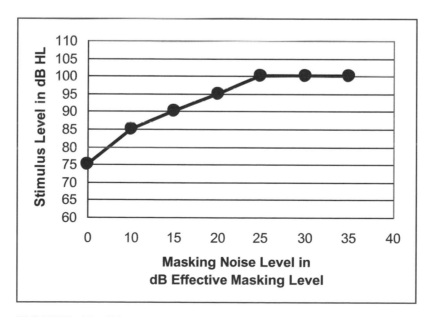

**FIGURE 13–27.** Patient response level as a function of presentation level of masking noise. There is no change in threshold with higher masking noise intensity.

neural hearing loss, overmasking would not occur until you have put at least 170 dB EML of masking noise in the nontest ear. This is, of course, well above the intensity limits of the equipment output. The areas of undermasking and effective masking for this example are demonstrated graphically in Figure 13–29.

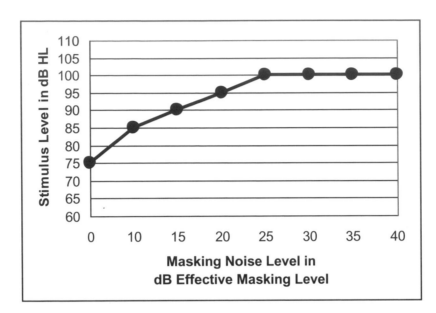

**FIGURE 13–28.** Patient response level as a function of presentation level of masking noise. There is no change in threshold with higher masking noise intensity. The stability of threshold suggests that this is an area of effect masking level.

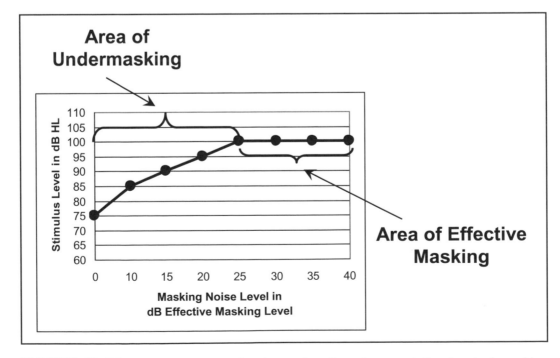

**FIGURE 13–29.** Patient response level as a function of presentation level of masking noise. Areas of undermasking and effective masking are labeled.

You record your masked air-conduction threshold on the audiogram using the appropriate symbol, as shown in Figure 13–30 and move on to obtain masked thresholds for the other frequencies.

To continue our example, imagine that you have completed the masked air-conduction audiogram for the right ear and have obtained the audiogram shown in Figure 13–31.

Now the bone-conduction thresholds must be considered. It is currently unknown whether the hearing loss in the right ear is conductive, mixed, or sensorineural. The left ear must be masked to determine accurate bone-conduction thresholds for the right ear. Once again, you will use the plateau method and begin with 1000 Hz. Narrowband noise will be presented to the left ear to cover up the signal being heard in the left ear. At what intensity level should the noise be presented? The air-conduction threshold in the left ear is 0 dB HL. Using the plateau method, add 10 dB EML of masking noise to the nontest ear air-conduction threshold. Why the air-conduction threshold? Because masking noise is presented via air conduction. So, begin by presenting 10 dB EML of masking noise to the left ear. After reestablishing threshold, it is found that the bone-conduction threshold has shifted to 20 dB HL as shown in the graph in Figure 13–32.

Following the plateau method, you then add another 5 dB EML to the masking noise. You reestablish the bone-conduction threshold in the right ear and find that it shifts another 5 dB as shown in Figure 13–33.

This process is repeated again and again. Each time, the intensity of the bone-conduction threshold increases. Masking noise level is increased until a test presentation level of 70 dB HL is reached. At this point, the patient does not respond to the bone-conducted signal at the

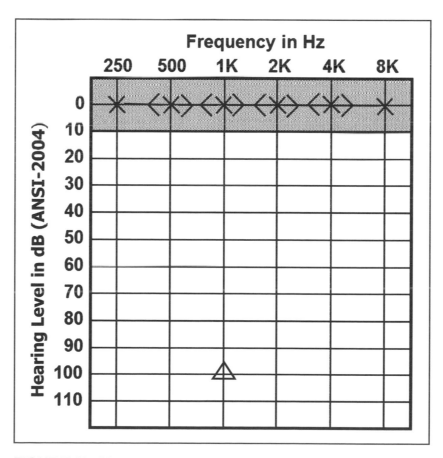

**FIGURE 13–30.** Audiogram showing addition of masked right ear air-conduction threshold.

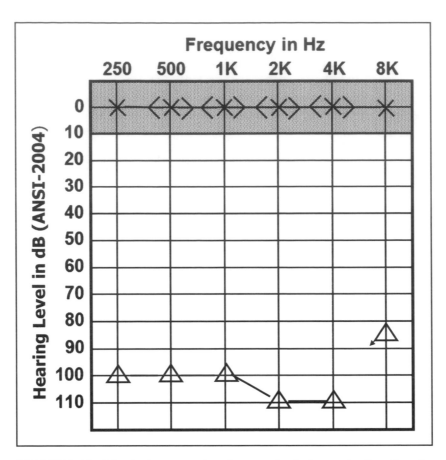

**FIGURE 13–31.** Audiogram showing masked air-conduction thresholds for the right ear.

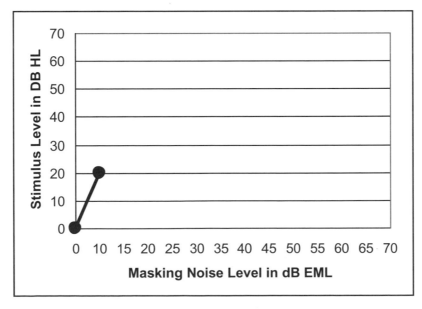

**FIGURE 13–32.** Patient response level as a function of presentation level of masking noise. There is a shift in threshold with addition of masking noise.

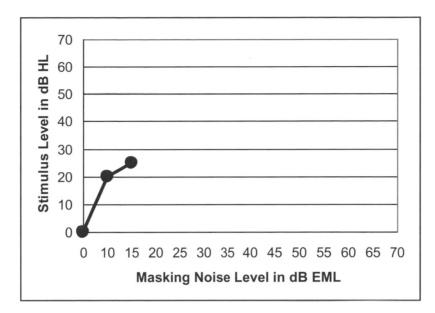

**FIGURE 13–33.** Patient response level as a function of presentation level of masking noise. There is an additional shift in threshold with higher masking noise intensity. The additional threshold shift suggests that this is an area of undermasking.

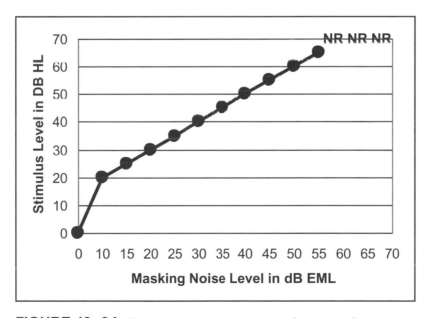

**FIGURE 13–34.** Patient response level as a function of presentation level of masking noise. There are additional shifts in threshold with higher masking noise until no response (NR) is observed.

limits of the bone-conductor output. This occurs as masking noise level is increased further, as is shown in Figure 13–34.

At this point, where there is no response at equipment limits, an effective masking level has been reached, as is shown in Figure 13–35.

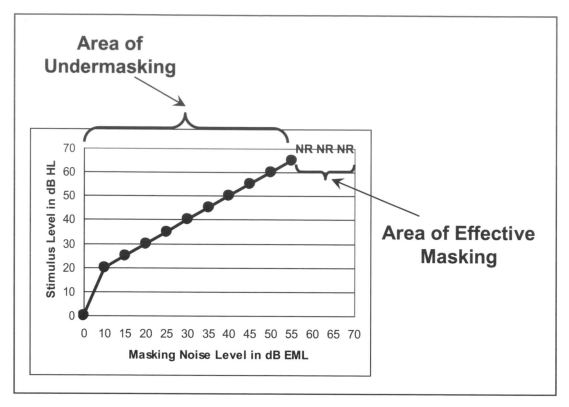

**FIGURE 13–35.** Patient response level as a function of presentation level of masking noise. Areas of undermasking and effective masking are labeled. (NR, no response.)

It is known that the level of masking is not overmasking, because the presentation level of the masking noise is below the level of minimum interaural attenuation for an insert earphone. Because the bone-vibrator transducer is limited to a level of output less than that of the air-conduction transducer, it is technically impossible to know whether the patient has a mixed versus a sensorineural hearing loss. Immittance information must be utilized to further understand the type of hearing loss. However, a pure conductive hearing loss has been ruled out for the right ear. After obtaining all of the masked bone-conduction thresholds, the results would be noted on the audiogram as shown in Figure 13–36.

Consider another example. Imagine that the unmasked audiogram shown in Figure 13–37 was obtained using supra-aural earphones.

As can be seen in Table 13–1, minimum interaural attenuation values for supra-aural earphones are lower than for insert earphones. The unmasked air-conduction thresholds for the right ear potentially could have been the result of being heard by crossover in the left ear. To determine whether this was the case, masking for air-conduction is necessary.

Using the plateau method, 10 dB EML of masking noise is placed into the left ear with narrowband noise centered at 1000 Hz. (This is 10 dB greater than the air-conduction threshold for the left ear.) Threshold is then reestablished for the right ear. There is no change in the patient's threshold as is shown in Figure 13–38.

The intensity of the masker noise is then raised by 5 dB EML, and threshold is reestablished. Again, there is no change in the patient response. Once again, the masking noise level is increased by 5 dB EML and threshold is reestablished, and again, there is no change in threshold, as shown in Figure 13–39.

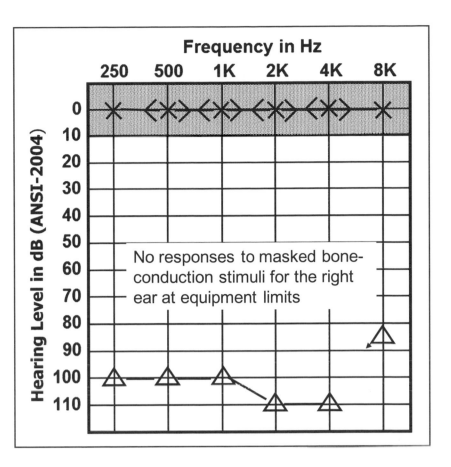

**FIGURE 13–36.** Audiogram showing addition of information regarding masked bone-conduction responses for the right ear.

No responses to masked bone-conduction stimuli for the right ear at equipment limits

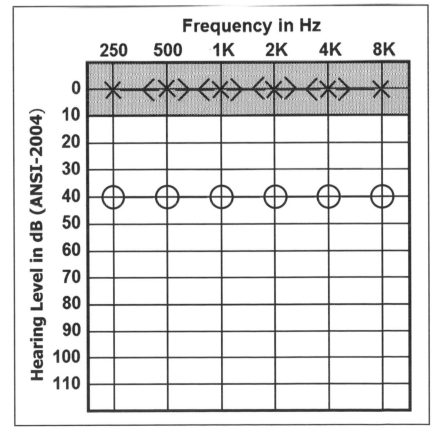

**FIGURE 13–37.** Unmasked air- and bone- conduction thresholds for the left and right ears.

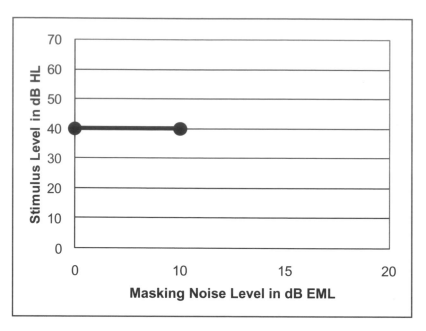

**FIGURE 13–38.** Patient response level as a function of presentation level of masking noise. Despite increasing the intensity of the masking noise, the threshold remains stable.

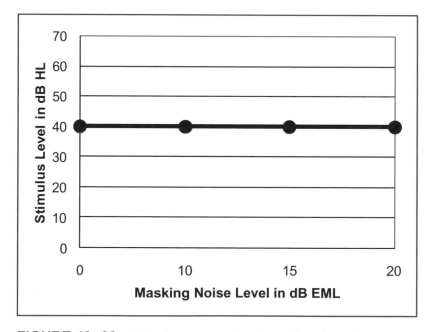

**FIGURE 13–39.** Patient response level as a function of presentation level of masking noise. Despite increasing the intensity of the masking noise, the threshold remains stable over several trials, demonstrating a plateau from which it can be determined that an effective masking level is being used and that the patient response represents the true threshold.

The lack of change in the threshold with masking noise demonstrates that the unmasked air-conduction threshold is correct. To demonstrate that masking was utilized to obtain the threshold, the symbol recorded on the audiogram is changed to a masked, right ear air-conduction symbol. This process is repeated for the remaining frequencies, and it is determined that the thresholds remained stable. The resulting audiogram is shown in Figure 13–40.

Next, the accuracy of the unmasked bone-conduction thresholds needs to be evaluated. The unmasked bone-conduction thresholds for the right ear potentially could have been the result of being heard by crossover in the left ear. To determine whether this was the case, masking for bone conduction is necessary.

Using the plateau method, 10 dB EML of masking noise is placed into the left ear with narrowband noise centered at 1000 Hz. (This is 10 dB greater than the air-conduction threshold for the left ear.) Threshold is then reestablished for the right ear. It is found that the bone-conduction threshold shifts to 20 dB HL as shown in Figure 13–41. The intensity of the masker noise is then raised by 5 dB EML, and threshold is reestablished.

The bone-conduction threshold shifts by 5 dB to 25 dB HL. This process is repeated until, with 35 dB EML of masking noise, the threshold remains stable at 40 dB HL as shown in Figure 13–42.

You continue to increase the EML until the threshold has been stable for three consecutive trials, indicating that an effective masking level has been achieved. In this example, this occurs at a test signal intensity of 40 dB HL. For the purposes of our example, imagine that you continued to increase the level of the masking noise. The masker intensity is increased over multiple trials, and the threshold remains stable. However, when the masker intensity is increased again, the

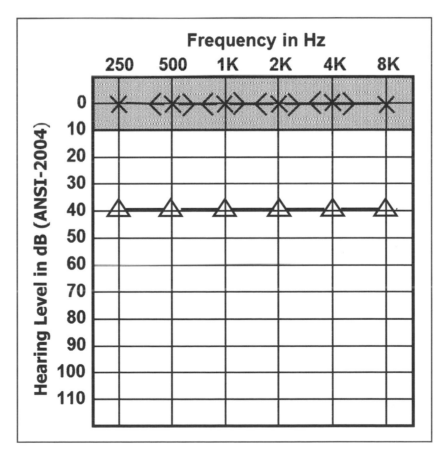

**FIGURE 13–40.** Audiogram showing addition of masked air-conduction thresholds for the right ear.

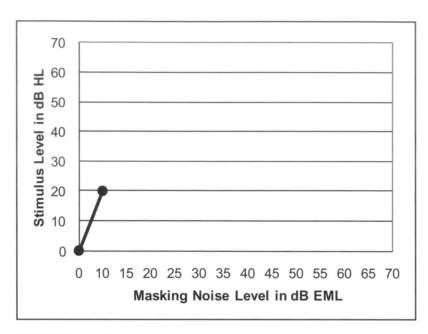

**FIGURE 13–41.** Patient response level as a function of presentation level of masking noise. There is a shift in threshold with addition of masking noise.

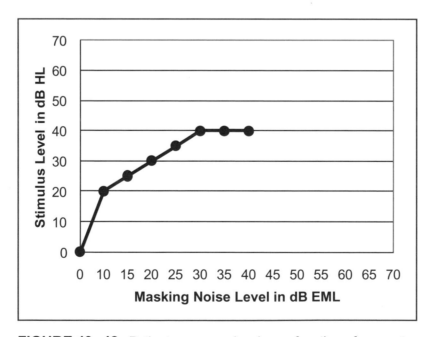

**FIGURE 13–42.** Patient response level as a function of presentation level of masking noise. The area of threshold shifts with increases in masking noise represents an area of undermasking. The area of threshold stability with increases in masking noise represents an area of effective masking.

reestablished threshold shifts by 5 dB HL. This continues over the next several trials as shown in Figure 13–43.

What has occurred that has caused a shift in the masked threshold? The answer is that overmasking has occurred. The masker noise is intense enough that it has crossed over by bone conduction to the test ear and is raising the threshold level of the test ear. This is why the reestablished threshold continued to rise in intensity. The areas of undermasking, effective masking, and overmasking are labeled in Figure 13–44.

The use of masking allowed you to determine that the masked bone-conduction threshold for the right ear was 40 dB HL. The process was repeated for the other frequencies and the thresholds plotted as shown in Figure 13–45. The use of masking allowed the clinician to determine that the hearing loss in the right ear was sensorineural in nature.

## Cases When Masking Does Not Work

There are a few instances where you will find yourself unable to use masking techniques to establish a valid threshold for a given ear.

### Equipment Intensity Limits

When the amount of masking noise required to establish a valid masked threshold exceeds the intensity limits of the audiometer, you simply cannot make the masking sound intense enough. In the example audiogram shown in Figure 13–46, there is a profound hearing loss bilaterally. For most audiometers, the maximum output level for masking noise is lower than the level for puretone output. Unmasked bone-conduction thresholds are present in the moderately severe region. Despite the fact that the bone vibrator was on the right mastoid, due to the minimal interaural

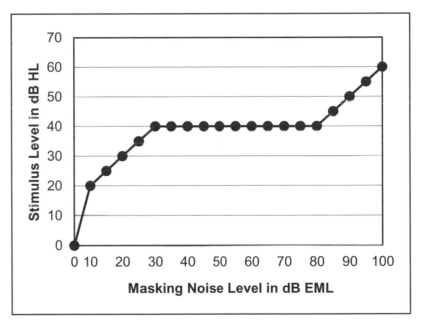

**FIGURE 13–43.** Patient response level as a function of presentation level of masking noise. The area of threshold shifts with increases in masking noise represents an area of undermasking. The area of threshold stability with increases in masking noise represents an area of effective masking. The area of threshold shifts with increases in masking noise beyond effective masking represents an area of overmasking.

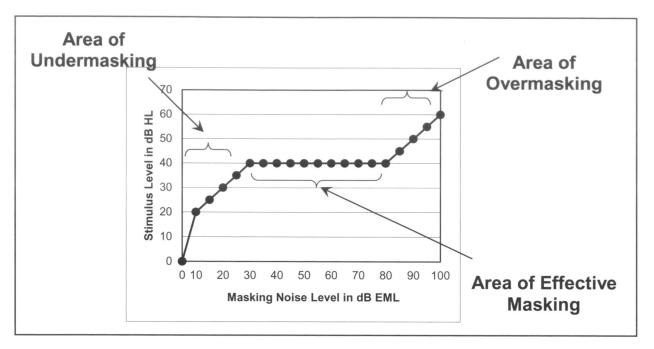

FIGURE 13-44. Patient response level as a function of presentation level of masking noise. Areas of undermasking, effective masking, and overmasking are labeled.

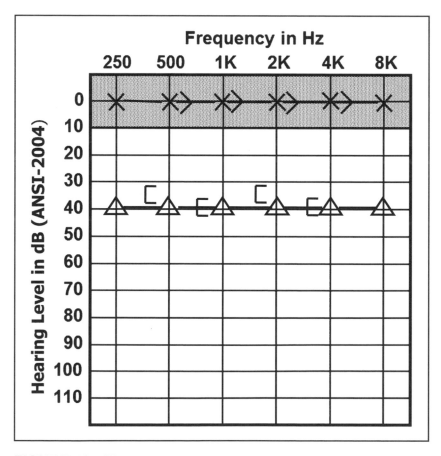

FIGURE 13-45. Audiogram showing addition of masked bone-conduction thresholds for the right ear.

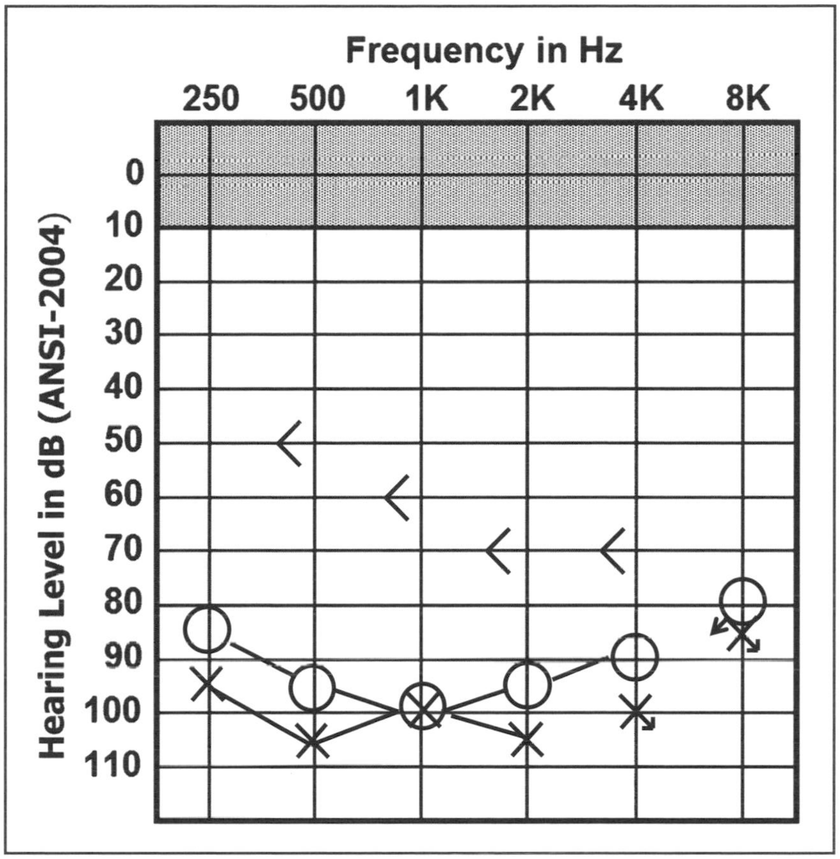

**FIGURE 13–46.** Audiogram demonstrating thresholds that would create a situation where masking would not be likely to be able to be performed because the masking noise intensity is too low to mask, due to equipment limits on intensity.

attenuation of signals generated by the bone vibrator, we do not know whether the perception of these signals occurred in the right ear, the left ear, or some combination of the two. The audiologist would be forced to rely on other measures, such as immittance, to further understand the loss of function in this case.

*Clinical Note:* When the intensity of the bone vibrator becomes very high, a person may feel the vibration rather than hear it. For example, in the case of complete hearing loss in an ear, the patient may respond to the bone vibration at very high intensities because they are feeling the vibration rather than hearing the sound. Because sound is created by vibration, it may be difficult for some people to distinguish between what is heard and what is felt. You will need to be aware of this when interpreting the results of behavioral responses to high-intensity bone-conduction stimuli. Immittance and other measures can be helpful in such situations to understand the entire clinical presentation.

### Masking Dilemma

A problem known as the "masking dilemma" occurs when there is a substantial conductive component to hearing loss in both ears that does not allow a plateau to occur in the masking function. Basically, by the time enough masking has been introduced to overcome undermasking, overmasking has begun to occur. This is a dilemma because there is no opportunity to observe the occurrence of the plateau and to determine the level of effective masking.

Imagine that you are testing a patient using supra-aural earphones. You obtain the audiogram shown in Figure 13–47.

Although you have the bone vibrator placed on the right mastoid, you do not know whether the response is coming from the right cochlea or the left cochlea. You know you have a conductive hearing loss in at least one ear, but you do not know which ear that is. You also do not know whether there is a conductive, mixed, or sensorineural loss in the other ear. These are important things to know, and you would like to mask to find out the answers. Assume that you choose one ear to present masking noise. Imagine that you present masking noise in the left ear for 1000 Hz. Following the plateau method, you present an intensity of 10 dB greater than the air-conduction threshold for that ear (that is 65 dB EML of masking noise: 55 dB HL threshold + 10 dB EML of masking noise). Now, your bone-conduction threshold shifts by 10 dB. So you add another 5 dB EML of masking noise, and the threshold shifts by 5 dB. You continue this process over and over, and you continually observe that the threshold shifts every time you put in masking noise, as shown in Figure 13–48. You have no idea what this means.

The problem is that from the first trial, you have delivered 65 dB EML of masking noise into the left ear, which is greater than the minimum interaural attenuation value for supra-aural earphones at 1000 Hz (40 dB). You may have been overmasking from the first trial. Or you may have been undermasking and then gone straight into overmasking. There is no way to tell. You must rely on other methods of assessment to help you to understand the loss of function in the auditory system. Note that a masking dilemma is less likely to occur using insert earphones than when using supra-aural earphones, due to the increased interaural attenuation of insert earphones.

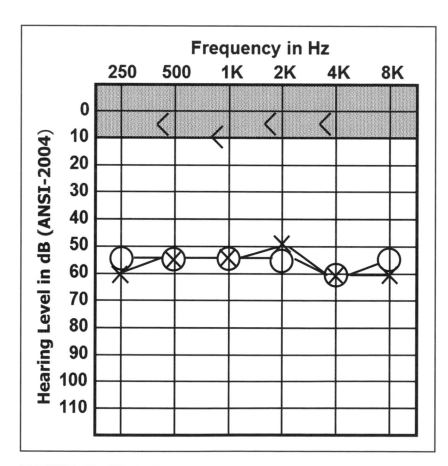

**FIGURE 13–47.** Audiogram demonstrating a masking dilemma for supra-aural earphones. The intensity level required to be an effective masking level would likely create a situation resulting in overmasking.

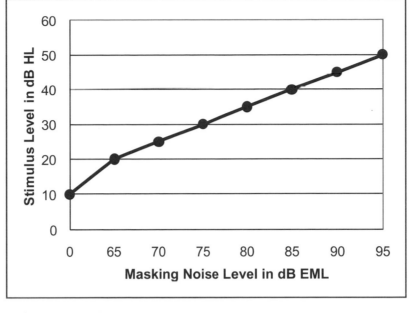

**FIGURE 13–48.** Patient response level as a function of presentation level of masking noise. Each additional increase in masking intensity results in an increase in threshold level. No plateau of effective masking level is observed. This phenomenon is called a *masking dilemma*.

## Occlusion Effect

Once you understand the plateau method for masking, you can consider a method to make the process more efficient. When the ear canal is occluded with an earphone (as you would need to do to introduce masking noise), the bone-conduction thresholds are artificially reduced, and appear better, by up to 10 dB. This phenomenon is known as the occlusion effect. Because the occlusion effect is predictable, we can account for the known enhancement of bone-conduction signals by modifying the initial presentation level for the masking noise. Rather than starting at 10 dB above the air-conduction threshold, you can add an additional amount of intensity to the initial masking noise. For 250 and 500 Hz, add 20 dB. For 1000 Hz, add 5 dB. So for the initial masking level, if you account for the occlusion effect, you would use 30 dB + the air-conduction threshold of the nontest ear for 250 and 500 Hz, and you would use 15 dB + the air-conduction threshold of the nontest ear for 1000 Hz.

When using the plateau method, correcting for occlusion effect when choosing a starting level is essentially a "shortcut." If you choose to follow the plateau method and ignore the occlusion effect, you will get to the plateau eventually. However, in the long run, this will be costly in terms of time and patient convenience.

## Additional Shortcuts

In most situations, it is possible to mask when performing air- and bone-conduction threshold testing and you cannot go wrong by masking. However, it is not always absolutely necessary to do so. In some cases, such as a busy clinical situation, the extra time needed to mask can be burdensome. Masking also can be difficult and/ or fatiguing to some patients. In cases where masking is not absolutely necessary, there may be legitimate reasons to forego masking and utilize unmasked thresholds. The following section describes situations when masking is not absolutely necessary.

When there is a possibility that the test signal can be heard in the nontest ear, you always need to mask. If you are testing via bone conduction, theoretically you always need to mask because the minimum interaural attenuation will always be 0 dB, and the test signal being presented is almost always greater than 0 dB HL. However, there is some "clinical leeway" in determining when to mask for bone conduction. The purpose of obtaining bone-conduction thresholds in a clinical situation is to determine whether the hearing loss is conductive, sensorineural, or mixed. Because of expected variation due test/retest reliability, there can be up to a 10 dB difference between bone-conduction and air-conduction thresholds before we begin to consider that there may be a conductive component to the hearing loss. If there is no "significant" air-bone gap (greater than 10 dB), then we can consider the hearing loss to be sensorineural, and masking is not necessary. For example, in the audiogram shown in Figure 13–49, the

bone vibrator was placed on the right and left mastoids, and all thresholds were obtained without masking noise.

Even though we do not technically know which ear the bone-conduction responses were originating from, there is no significant difference between the bone-conduction responses and the air-conduction responses (no air-bone gaps ≥10 dB). Therefore, we already know that there is no conductive hearing loss, so masking is not necessary. Remember that the threshold obtained by bone conduction is a result of the sensitivity of the cochlea. The threshold obtained by air conduction is from the outer ear, middle ear, and cochlea combined. If there is no pathology in the outer or middle ear, the air-conduction thresholds should approximately equal the bone-conduction thresholds. If there is pathology in the outer or middle ear

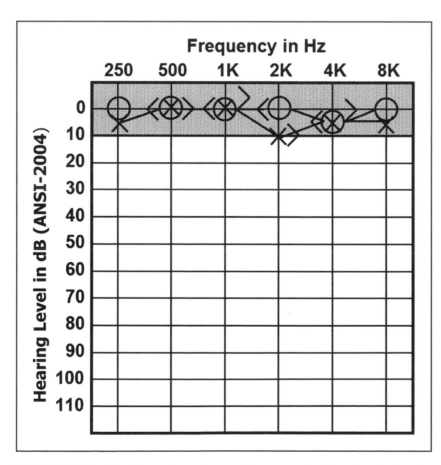

**FIGURE 13–49.** Unmasked air- and bone-conduction thresholds for the left and right ears. Masking is not absolutely necessary in this situation because there are no significant air-bone gaps.

that impacts function, the air-conduction thresholds are likely to be worse than the bone-conduction thresholds. In general, it can be assumed that bone-conduction thresholds will be the same as, or better than, air-conduction thresholds, and not worse than air-conduction thresholds.

To review, the purpose of masking is to prevent cross hearing of a signal that is intense enough to cross over to the nontest ear via bone conduction by introduction of masking noise into the nontest ear. The clinical utility of this strategy is to differentiate among conductive, mixed, and sensorineural hearing losses. When the signal presented is of sufficient intensity to be heard by crossover in the nontest ear, masking should be used to eliminate the potential for the patient to respond based on hearing the sound in the nontest ear.

## OBSERVATION

1. Observe an experienced clinician obtain pure-tone unmasked thresholds for a patient or volunteer.

2. Observe the clinician using the plateau method to find masked threshold. What types of instructions does the clinician give to the listener? Why do you think that appropriate instructions are so important for obtaining accurate thresholds?

_____

_____

_____

3. Does the clinician use a charting method to determine threshold, or is this process accomplished "in the head" of the clinician?

_____

## GUIDED PRACTICE

For Items 1, 2, 3, and 4 of the Guided Practice exercises, you may use the audiograms provided in Figures 13–50, 13–51, and 13–52.

1. Obtain an unmasked pure-tone audiogram on a volunteer on the first audiogram form.

2. Place a foam sound-attenuating earplug in one ear of a patient or volunteer. Using supra-aural earphones, obtain an unmasked pure-tone air- and bone-conduction audiogram for a patient or volunteer. Mark your responses with the appropriate symbols on the second audiogram form.

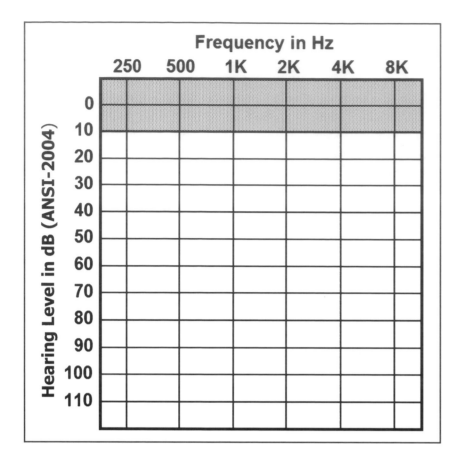

**FIGURE 13–50.** Audiogram for Guided Practice exercise.

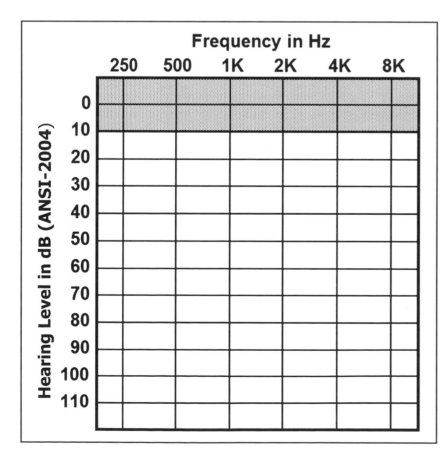

**FIGURE 13–51.** Audiogram for Guided Practice exercise.

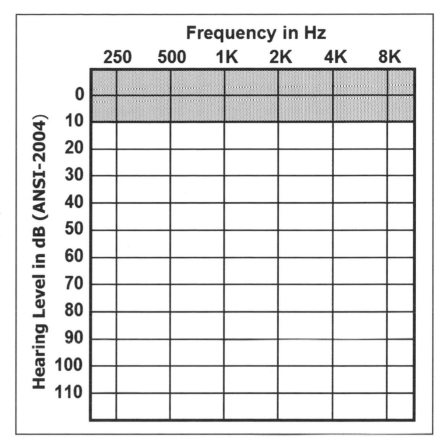

**FIGURE 13–52.** Audiogram for Guided Practice exercise.

3. Keeping the earplug in the ear, obtain masked thresholds for bone conduction. Mark your responses with the appropriate symbols on the second audiogram form.

4. Place a foam sound attenuating earplug in the other ear as well. Using supra-aural earphones, attempt to obtain masked bone-conduction thresholds. Mark your responses with the appropriate symbols on the third audiogram form. You may or may not be able to find a plateau level. What factors would influence your ability or inability to obtain a plateau level?

## REFLECTION AND REVIEW

1. The term for the ear that is being tested is

_____

2. The term for the ear that is not being tested is

_____

3. When sound is intense enough to stimulate the nontest ear, this is called

_____

4. Crossover happens via

_____

5. When sound that crosses over to the nontest ear is more intense than the bone-conduction threshold of that ear, what phenomenon occurs?

_____

6. What is the purpose of masking?

_____

_____

7. True or false: When using a masker, the test signal does not stimulate the nontest ear. Explain your answer.

_____

_____

8. What is the interaural attenuation in Figure 13–53?

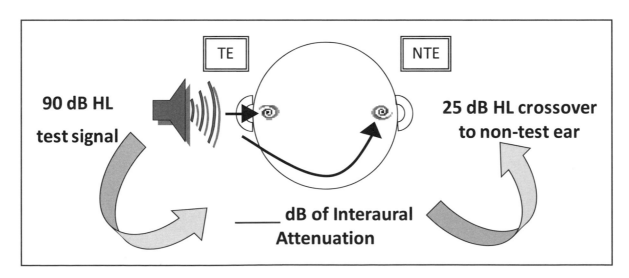

**FIGURE 13–53.** Concept of interaural attenuation.

_____

9. Assume that in the scenario shown in Figure 13–54, the patient's bone-conduction threshold for the nontest ear is 5 dB HL. Is the test signal heard by the patient in the nontest ear?

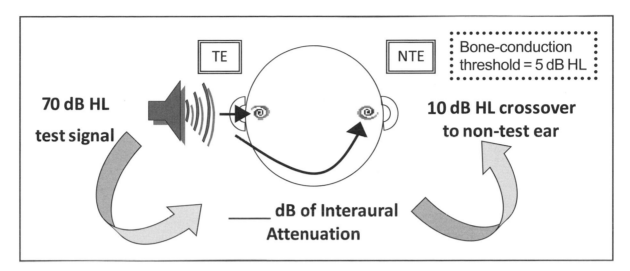

**FIGURE 13–54.** Concept of cross hearing.

_____

10. Interaural attenuation is lowest for what type of transducer?

_____

11. Interaural attenuation is highest for what type of transducer?

_____

12. What type of transducer would you use to minimize the possibility of a masking dilemma? Why?

_____

_____

13. What is undermasking?

_____

_____

14. What is overmasking?

_____

_____

15. What is the definition of the effective masking level?

_____

_____

# ||| 14 |||

## Speech Thresholds

### INTRODUCTION

Speech thresholds are used to determine a patient's sensitivity for either detecting or recognizing speech. Additionally, they are used to cross-check the validity of a patient's pure-tone thresholds and to provide a reference level for suprathreshold speech tests.

### LEARNING OUTCOMES

■ Understand some of the uses of the speech detection threshold (SDT)/speech awareness threshold (SAT).
■ Know how to obtain an SDT/SAT.
■ Be able to use an SDT/SAT to validate pure-tone thresholds.
■ Understand some of the uses of the speech reception (or recognition) threshold (SRT).
■ Know how to obtain an SRT.
■ Be able to use an SRT to validate pure-tone thresholds.

### REVIEW OF CONCEPTS

#### Speech Awareness Threshold/ Speech Detection Threshold

The speech detection threshold (SDT), also called the speech awareness threshold (SAT), is the lowest intensity level at which a patient demonstrates detection or awareness of speech. A speech detection threshold is obtained in a manner similar to pure-tone thresholds discussed in Chapter 10. Speech detection thresholds are determined by observing behavioral responses to speech sounds. This measure is most often used when testing young children but can be used with other populations as well, when speech recognition thresholds cannot be obtained.

To obtain the SDT/SAT with an adult or older child, the audiologist would ask the patient to respond anytime that speech is heard. This response could be raising the hand, saying "Yes," or pushing a button. When conducting this testing with young children or those with cognitive delays (such as infants and toddlers or special populations), the audiologist looks for behavioral responses such as head turn, eye gaze changes, or other behavioral responses. The audiologist presents a running speech signal (such as "ba ba ba" or the patient's name) via monitored live voice (MLV), which is carefully controlled using the VU meter on the audiometer.

The objective is to determine the lowest intensity level at which the signal is heard. This can be achieved in an ascending manner, initially presenting the signal well below the anticipated response level and raising the intensity of the signal in 5 dB steps. As soon as the patient responds, the audiologist lowers the intensity level and begins the process of obtaining threshold using the modified Hughson-Westlake technique, determining the level at which the patient hears the signal 50% of the time. Remember, when presenting the signal via monitored live voice, it is critical that the patient not see the audiologist, or at least not be able to see the lips or face of the audiologist.

## Speech Recognition Threshold

The speech recognition threshold (SRT) is the lowest intensity level at which a patient demonstrates the ability to identify speech 50% of the time. Identification typically is assessed by repetition of words. This can be done through other methods such as pointing to pictures.

The words used for determining SRTs are known as *spondees*. Spondees are two-syllable words that have equal stress on each syllable. Examples are words such as baseball, cowboy, hot dog, sidewalk, airplane, playground, ice cream, popcorn, football, and cupcake.

The use of monitored live voice (MLV) versus use of recorded materials has been found to have little effect on the outcomes of speech threshold testing. Because of this determination, and because the use of MLV is more efficient for establishing SRT, MLV is typically the chosen method. However, in cases where the tester has speech that may be perceived as heavily accented relative to that of the tested population, recorded materials should be used. To use monitored live voice, the tester must present words at a consistent intensity level. The tester must monitor the input by examination of the VU meter on the audiometer to ensure that speech stimuli are neither too loud nor too soft. It is common practice to utilize a carrier phrase such as "Say the word . . . " prior to presentation of the spondee, although this is not always performed.

Because patients may perform more poorly if they are unfamiliar with a particular word, it is good practice to familiarize the patient with the word list prior to initiating testing. This can be accomplished by finding a comfortable listening level and presenting the words to the patient at this level. Once the patient has had the opportunity to repeat the words at a comfortable level, the intensity can be reduced for the purpose of determining the threshold level. Again, it is crucial that the patient not see the face of the audiologist during this testing, if it is conducted using monitored live voice. Therefore, the audiologist must either be out of view of the patient, or must completely cover her or his face to avoid presentation of any visual speech cues.

The threshold level can be determined by first presenting the words at a comfortable level, to familiarize the listener with the word list. The level is then decreased to 30 dB HL and a single word is presented. If the patient responds correctly at 30 dB HL, the intensity is decreased by 10 dB. This process is continued with presentation of a single word until the patient fails to respond or responds incorrectly. If the patient does not respond or responds incorrectly at 30 dB HL, the intensity is increased by 20 dB. This process is continued with presentation of a single word until the patient responds correctly. Once the initial level is determined, the tester presents up to five words. If the patient correctly responds to fewer than three words, the intensity should be increased by 5 dB. If the patient identifies three or more words, the intensity should be decreased by 10 dB. The lowest intensity level at which the patient correctly repeats at least three of five words correctly is the speech reception threshold.

## Relationships Among Speech Recognition Thresholds, Speech Detection Thresholds, and the Audiogram

Because speech is used to determine speech thresholds, the thresholds of the pure-tone frequencies that are most important for speech understanding should closely match the SRT. Specifically, an average of the pure-tone thresholds at 500, 1000, and 2000 Hz (known as the pure-tone average or PTA) should match the SRT within 7 to 10 dB. When SRT measures do not closely match the PTA (with the SRT measure tending to be lower in intensity than the PTA) this may indicate functional or exaggerated hearing loss. There are exceptions to the rule that the SRT and PTA should closely match, such as in cases of highly configured losses. For example, if 500 and 1000 Hz thresholds are 20 dB HL, but hearing at 2000 Hz drops to 80 dB HL, the SRT would likely be close to 20 dB HL, rather than the PTA of 40 dB HL.

Regarding the speech detection threshold, the intensity level of the SDT should correspond to the lowest intensity level of the pure-tone frequencies tested, rather than the PTA.

## OBSERVATION

1. Observe an experienced clinician obtain a speech awareness threshold for a patient or volunteer.

2. Observe the clinician obtain a speech recognition threshold for a patient or volunteer.

## GUIDED PRACTICE

1. Prepare a volunteer for speech threshold testing. Explain to the listener what you would like them to do.

2. Obtain a speech detection threshold for a volunteer.

3. Obtain a speech recognition threshold for a volunteer.

4. Obtain pure-tone thresholds on the same volunteer and calculate the pure-tone average. How does the PTA compare to the SDT and the SRT?

## REFLECTION AND REVIEW

1. What are the three main purposes of speech threshold testing?

_____

_____

_____

2. Provide the definition of the pure-tone average.

_____

3. Provide the definition of the speech recognition threshold.

_____

4. What is a spondee?

_____

5. What instructions would you provide to a patient to obtain an SRT?

_____

_____

_____

6. Explain why the pure-tone average of 500, 1000, and 2000 Hz should closely match the SRT.

_____

_____

7. Describe circumstances when you may wish to obtain speech detection thresholds rather than speech recognition thresholds.

_____

_____

8. Describe how to use the VU meter to perform monitored live voice testing for determining speech thresholds.

_____

_____

_____

9.  If the SRT is significantly lower than the PTA, what would this indicate to you about the validity of the patient's responses?

    _____

    _____

    _____

# ▌▌▌ 15 ▌▌▌

## Word Recognition Testing

### INTRODUCTION

Word recognition testing is a valuable component of the audiometric evaluation. This testing is performed at a suprathreshold level. Word recognition testing can be used for a number of purposes including provision of diagnostic information, assessment of suprathreshold speech understanding, and cross-check of pure-tone sensitivity.

### LEARNING OUTCOMES

- Understand the purposes of word recognition testing.
- Know how to perform word recognition testing.
- Understand the performance-intensity function derived from word recognition testing.

### REVIEW OF CONCEPTS

#### Purposes of Word Recognition Testing

There are several reasons why word recognition testing is performed. An important function of word recognition testing is its potential value as a diagnostic indicator. Typically, word recognition performance can be predicted by the audiogram. However, in some cases, such as when there is central auditory or retrocochlear dysfunction, word recognition scores may be poorer than expected, alerting the clinician to the possibility of these problems.

Word recognition testing also can be used as an assessment of suprathreshold speech understanding. When considering rehabilitation measures, it is helpful to have knowledge of how a patient understands speech when sound is made loud enough to hear well. Individuals who have poor word recognition at suprathreshold levels should be counseled as to appropriate expectations for amplification.

Another use of word recognition testing is as a cross-check of pure-tone sensitivity. If word recognition scores are dramatically better than should be expected for a given audiogram, this may be an indication of functional hearing loss. In addition, if word recognition scores are high at a very low sensation level relative to the speech reception (or recognition) threshold (SRT), this can also raise concern about functional hearing loss.

#### Performing Word Recognition Testing

Word recognition testing is performed by presenting open-set monosyllabic words (words of one syllable) at a fixed intensity level that is audible to the patient. The patient repeats back the word that is presented. The percentage of correct responses is calculated.

## Test Materials

Most word recognition lists are 50 words in length. The lists of words typically used are grouped so that they are phonetically balanced, meaning that the speech sounds present in the lists occur with the same frequency as those found in conversational speech in English. Numerous word lists are available, including the Harvard Psychoacoustics Lab PAL PB-50, the Central Institute for the Deaf CID W-22, and the Northwestern University NU-6. Most tests have published norms to determine expected versus abnormal scores. When reporting results, the clinician should provide information about the specific word list used to obtain results.

## Presentation Method

The two methods available for presentation of stimuli are monitored live voice and recorded materials. In all situations, recorded materials are the method of choice for stimulus presentation. The use of recorded materials allows comparison of test scores between presenters, between test sessions, and with normative data. Without the ability to compare word recognition scores in this manner, the resulting test data would rarely, if ever, be useful for any purpose.

Typically, a carrier phrase is presented, followed by the stimulus. An example is, "Say the word 'wife'." The patient then responds by repeating the last word of the sentence.

## Presentation Level

Performance on tests of word recognition depends to a certain extent on the audibility of speech sounds. In other words, the sounds must be loud enough to be heard. It has been found that, for most normal hearing listeners, the maximum speech recognition performance occurs at a level of about 40 dB greater than the speech recognition threshold (40 dB sensation level, re: SRT). However, depending on the configuration of the hearing loss, some sounds may still be inaudible.

The most efficient strategy for obtaining maximum word recognition performance scores is to present words at a high intensity level, for example, 80 dB HL. For most listeners, this will allow nearly all speech sounds to be audible, and the maximum score for performance can be quickly obtained.

The use of high-intensity levels for presentation of word recognition stimuli is also beneficial for diagnostic purposes, such as determining whether rollover is occurring.

## Performance-Intensity Function and Rollover

For most individuals with normal auditory function or purely cochlear hearing loss, maximum word recognition performance is maintained at high intensity levels. The term *rollover* is used to describe the phenomenon of decreased word recognition ability with increasing intensity levels. This phenomenon often is observed in cases of retrocochlear pathology, and therefore can be used as a diagnostic indicator.

The presence of rollover can be observed by testing word recognition performance at a number of different intensity levels. The resulting performance can be plotted to obtain a performance-intensity function. A performance-intensity function is a graph of the percentage correct speech score as a function of the presentation level. Such a graph can help the clinician to determine whether performance is normal or whether rollover is occurring. Figure 15–1A demonstrates a normal performance-intensity function. Figure 15–1B demonstrates rollover observed on a performance-intensity function.

The initial use of a high intensity level becomes efficient when thinking about the use of word recognition testing for diagnostic purposes. By using a high intensity level, the tester is essen-

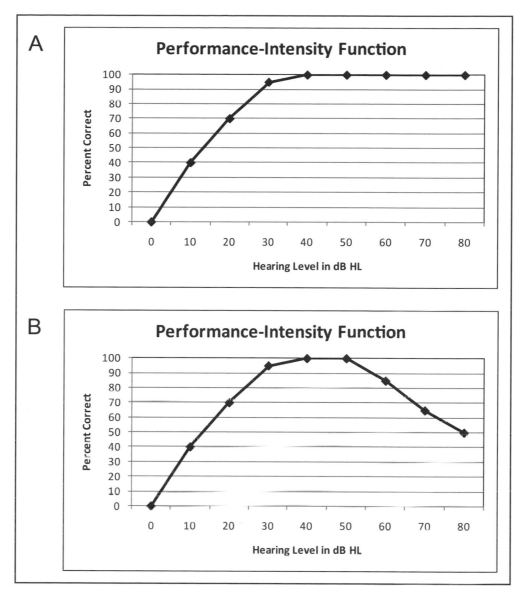

**FIGURE 15–1. A.** A normal performance-intensity function. Percentage correct on word recognition testing as a function of presentation level in dB HL. **B.** Rollover observed on a performance-intensity function. At the highest intensity presentation level, word recognition performance decreases relative to lower intensity levels.

tially "beginning at the end" of the performance-intensity function. If a patient performs optimally as predicted (according to published norms) at the high intensity level, then rollover is not occurring. If a patient performs less than optimally at the high intensity level, then the tester is cued to the possibility that rollover may be occurring and

that lower intensity levels should then be used to develop a performance-intensity function to evaluate this possibility. Figure 15–2 demonstrates the utility of first determining the performance at a high intensity level by showing how the highest intensity allows for determination of whether rollover is a possibility.

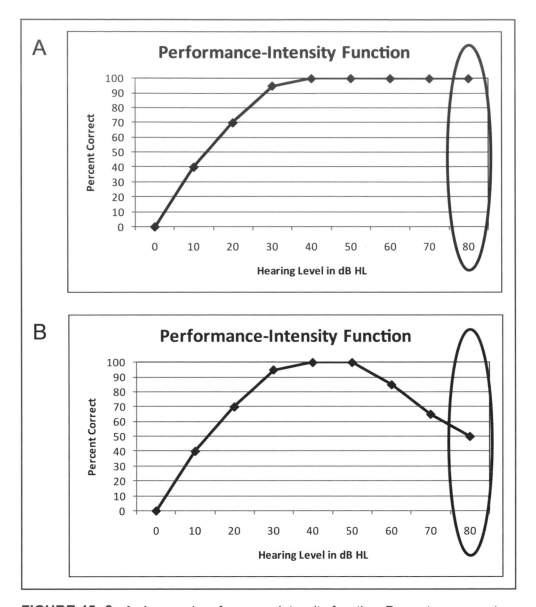

**FIGURE 15–2. A.** A normal performance-intensity function. Percentage correct on word recognition testing as a function of presentation level in dB HL. **B.** Rollover observed on a performance-intensity function. High intensity levels are highlighted to demonstrate that the value obtained at this level would allow the clinician to determine whether rollover is a possibility.

## OBSERVATION

1. Observe an experienced clinician obtain a word recognition score for a patient or volunteer.

2. Observe the clinician obtain a performance-intensity function for a patient or volunteer.

## GUIDED PRACTICE

For Items 2 and 3 of the Guided Practice exercises, you may use the Performance-Intensity Graphs in Figure 15–3, for the right and left ears.

1. Prepare a volunteer for word recognition testing. Provide instructions as to how the listener should respond.

2. Obtain a word recognition score using recorded speech materials at a level of 80 dB HL for a volunteer, for both the right and left ears.

3. Create a performance-intensity function by also obtaining word recognition scores at 70, 60, and 50 dB HL using different lists of recorded speech materials, for both the right and left ears.

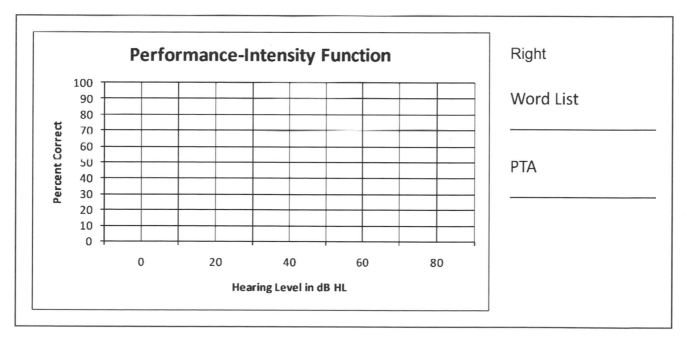

**FIGURE 15–3.** Performance-intensity graphs for right and left ears for Guided Practice exercise. *continues*

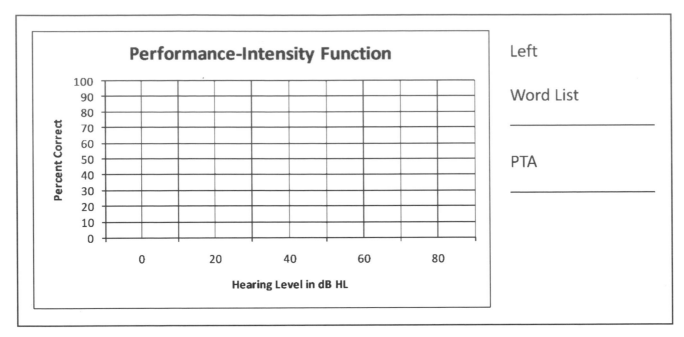

**FIGURE 15–3.** *continued*

## REFLECTION AND REVIEW

1. Explain the purposes of obtaining word recognition scores.

   _____

   _____

   _____

2. Describe the instructions that you would provide to a patient who is undergoing word recognition testing.

   _____

   _____

   _____

   _____

3. Describe the process of obtaining word recognition scores.

_____

_____

_____

_____

4. Describe the process of obtaining a performance-intensity function.

_____

_____

_____

5. Explain the necessity of using recorded speech materials.

_____

_____

_____

_____

6. What is rollover? Explain why it is important to determine whether rollover is occurring.

_____

_____

_____

_____

7. Explain the advantage of initially performing speech recognition testing at high intensity levels.

_____

_____

_____

_____

8. What would you suspect if your patient obtained high word recognition scores at low intensity levels if pure-tone thresholds demonstrate significant hearing loss?

_____

_____

9. Describe how word recognition testing is different than listening in a "real-world" situation. Why is this important to consider?

_____

_____

_____

_____

# III 16 III

## Masking for Speech Audiometry

### INTRODUCTION

Just as for pure-tone audiometry, masking is a necessary factor to consider when performing speech audiometry. The concepts for masking of speech are largely the same as those for pure tones but require an understanding of how the speech signal differs from pure tones.

### LEARNING OUTCOMES

■ Know when to mask for speech audiometry.
■ Know how to mask for speech audiometry.

### REVIEW OF CONCEPTS

When the sound in the test ear is sufficiently intense, it can vibrate the bones of the skull, causing the sound to stimulate the cochlea of the nontest ear. When the sound that reaches the nontest ear is greater than the bone-conduction threshold in the nontest ear, the sound can be heard by the patient.

Masking is the use of noise to prevent a test signal from being responded to when it is heard in the nontest ear. The goal of masking is to eliminate the ability of the nontest ear to "hear" the test signal by stimulating it with noise loud enough to disguise the test signal. If there is any chance that the test signal can be heard by crossover in the nontest ear, we need to mask so we know which ear we are actually testing. Refer to Chapter 13 for a review of general masking concepts.

Speech is a broadband signal. It is composed of many different frequencies. These different frequencies all have different levels of interaural attenuation. When masking for speech, the minimum interaural attenuation for the speech signal is the lowest level of interaural attenuation (IA) for speech-frequency pure tones. For supra-aural earphones, assume that minimum interaural attenuation may be as low as 40 dB HL. For insert earphones, assume that minimum interaural attenuation may be as low as 60 dB HL.

### When to Mask for Speech Recognition Threshold and Word Recognition Testing

First, consider that this is a challenging question because decisions regarding the need to mask may be dependent on the order of testing. The answers may be different depending on whether you know what the pure-tone air- and bone-conduction thresholds are prior to speech testing. In this chapter, the authors assume that the clinician has determined air- and bone-conduction thresholds for the patient before initiating any speech testing. This is done to assist the reader in the general concepts of masking for speech testing. However, in a clinical situation, you might test in a different order, with different masking procedures employed dependent on the order of the audiometry battery. This is completely acceptable, as long as masking is used appropriately, when necessary.

If the difference between the presentation level of the speech stimuli and the best pure-tone bone-conduction threshold of the contralateral ear is greater than or equal to minimum interaural attenuation for the earphone used, masking should be used. For supra-aural earphones, this minimum difference is 40 dB; for insert earphones it is 60 dB.

## Stimuli for Speech Audiometry Masking

Most two-channel audiometers have the option for speech-shaped noise as a masker. This noise is relatively broadband in nature. The signal is adjusted to mask the long-term spectrum of the speech signal.

## How to Mask for Speech Audiometry—Word Recognition

Determining the appropriate intensity level of noise in the nontest ear is crucial to avoid undermasking (too little noise, therefore allowing the nontest ear to participate in the test) or overmasking (too much noise, therefore crossing to the test ear). One process for masking of speech is the plateau method described in Chapter 13. Another approach to masking is to use a formula method. The advantage of this type of method is it quickly raises the masker intensity to an effective masking level. Several different formulae can be used for masking in speech audiometry; two are discussed below.

When testing word recognition, the following formula may be used (Yacullo, 1996):

Effective masking level =
Presentation level of the test ear − 20 dB

For example, when the presentation level of the test ear is 60 dB HL, the masking level used would be 40 dB HL. This formula generally can be used in cases without air-bone gaps (using the procedures for testing word recognition in Chapter 15), or when insert earphones are used. Note, however, that it is the tester's responsibility to always determine whether over- or undermasking might be occurring.

Consider the audiogram in Figure 16–1. Assume that you are going to present speech stimuli for word recognition testing at a level of 80 dB HL to the right ear, using insert earphones. At what level should the masker intensity be set for the left ear? The formula described above is appropriate for this situation because insert earphones are used for testing. The appropriate values should be applied to the formula shown above:

Effective masking level = 80 dB
(presentation level of the test ear) − 20 dB

In this case, 60 dB of masking should be used in the nontest (left) ear. When air-bone gaps are present, and when higher presentation levels are used with supra-aural earphones, the following formula is useful (Studebaker, 1979):

Effective masking level =
Presentation level of the test ear −
interaural attenuation + largest air-bone gap in
the nontest ear + a safety factor

This formula is recommended for the presence of the air-bone gaps, building in a safety factor to mask peak speech levels. *Note:* The safety factor may be up to 20 dB and may not always be necessary. The tester should use clinical judgment, especially when presenting speech signals at high intensity levels.

Again, consider the audiogram in Figure 16–1. Assume that you are going to present speech stim-

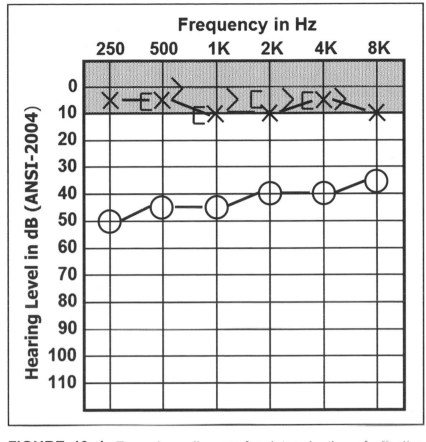

**FIGURE 16–1.** Example audiogram for determination of effective masking level for speech audiometry.

uli for word recognition testing at a level of 80 dB HL to the right ear, using supra-aural earphones. At what level should the masker intensity be set for the left ear? The second formula is useful in this situation because supra-aural earphones are used. To determine this level, the appropriate amounts should be applied to the formula shown above:

Effective masking level =
80 dB (presentation level of the test ear)
− 40 dB (interaural attenuation)
+ 5 dB (largest air-bone gap of the nontest ear)
+ up to 20 dB (safety factor)

In this case, the effective masking level could be as high as 65 dB. The tester should use clinical judgment, especially when presenting speech signals at high intensity levels.

## How to Mask for Speech Audiometry— Speech Recognition Threshold

The rules for when to mask are the same as for word recognition testing: If the difference between the presentation level of the speech stimuli and the best pure-tone bone conduction threshold of the contralateral ear is greater than or equal to minimum interaural attenuation for the transducer type, masking should be used.

One formula to determine the masking level is the one previously discussed:

Effective masking level =
Presentation level of the test ear − 20 dB

(Yacullo, 1996). The implementation will be slightly different, however. In this case, the presentation level is the highest level used during the

SRT test (typically 30–40 dB SL, re: the PTA when the clinician is familiarizing the listener with the words). Even though the clinician will decrease the intensity level for presentation during the SRT, it typically will not be necessary to reduce the masking level. When utilized during the SRT test, this formula may result in high masking levels. It is the clinician's responsibility to determine that overmasking has not occurred.

## OBSERVATION

1. Observe an experienced clinician obtain unmasked speech thresholds for a patient or volunteer.

2. Observe the clinician determine whether or not there is a need to mask for speech thresholds.

3. Observe the clinician reestablish speech threshold for a patient or volunteer using masking.

4. Observe the clinician obtain masked word recognition scores for a patient or volunteer.

## GUIDED PRACTICE

1. Obtain unmasked speech thresholds for a volunteer. Determine whether masking is necessary.

2. Place a foam sound attenuating earplug in one ear of the volunteer. Using supra-aural earphones, obtain unmasked speech thresholds for a patient or volunteer.

3. Keeping the earplug in the ear, obtain masked speech thresholds for a patient or volunteer.

4. Keeping the earplug in the ear, obtain unmasked word recognition scores for a patient or volunteer at 80 dB HL intensity level using supra-aural earphones. Is masking necessary in this case? Why or why not?

_____

_____

_____

_____

5. After obtaining unmasked thresholds, retest word recognition using masking in the nontest ear.

## REFLECTION AND REVIEW

1. What type of noise is used for masking in speech audiometry?

   _____

2. What is the purpose of masking?

   _____

   _____

   _____

3. Describe when masking should be used for speech threshold testing.

   _____

   _____

   _____

4. Describe when masking should be used for word recognition testing.

   _____

   _____

   _____

5. You have not yet tested bone conduction or performed immittance measures. Using supra-aural earphones, you find that your patient has an unmasked SRT in the left ear of 20 dB HL and in the right ear of 50 dB HL. Do you need to mask to ensure that your speech recognition thresholds are accurate? If so, which ear(s) do you need to mask? Why?

   _____

   _____

   _____

   _____

6. You have obtained immittance measurements for your patient and have found evidence of normal middle ear function bilaterally. Your unmasked SRTs using insert earphones are 40 dB HL bilaterally. Your presentation level for word recognition testing is 80 dB HL. Do you need to mask for word recognition testing? Why or why not?

_____

_____

_____

_____

# ||| 17 |||

## The Stenger Test

The Stenger test is a useful way to evaluate whether an individual demonstrating asymmetric thresholds has a nonorganic or exaggerated hearing loss. It can be used any time there is a 20 dB or greater difference between pure-tone or speech recognition thresholds between ears. The Stenger test also can be used to estimate an individual's actual threshold.

## LEARNING OUTCOMES

- Understand the Stenger effect.
- Understand the purpose of the Stenger test.
- Know when to use the Stenger test.
- Know how to administer the Stenger test.
- Understand the outcome of a Stenger test.
- Know how to estimate threshold with a Stenger test.

## REVIEW OF CONCEPTS

### The Stenger Effect

When a signal of the same phase and intensity is presented to a listener, the sound will be perceived only in the ear in which it is louder, or the ear with the higher sensation level (SL). Suppose a listener has a 10 dB HL threshold for a sound in the right ear and a 30 dB HL threshold for the same sound in the left ear as shown in Figure 17–1.

When the same signal is presented to both ears at the same time, in the same phase, and at the same intensity, it will be perceived in only the ear where there is a higher sensation level. Assume that you presented a 50 dB HL pure tone at the same time to both ears, as shown in Figure 17–2. The sensation level would be 40 dB SL in the right ear and 20 dB SL in the left ear. Due to the Stenger effect, the patient would perceive and report hearing the sound only in the right ear, the ear with the higher sensation level, as shown in Figure 17–3.

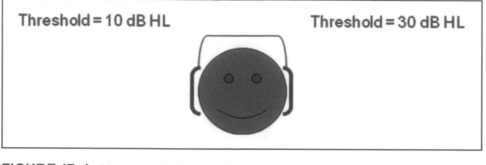

**FIGURE 17–1.** Listener with 20 dB difference between air-conduction thresholds.

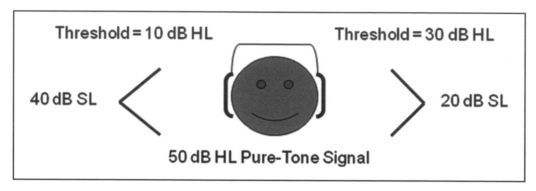

**FIGURE 17–2.** A 50 dB HL pure tone is presented to a patient with a 20 dB difference in threshold between ears resulting in different sensation levels in the ears.

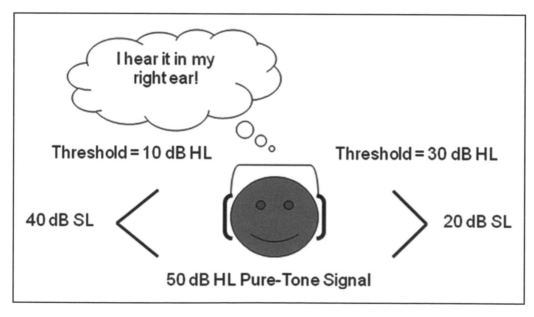

**FIGURE 17–3.** Demonstration of the Stenger effect. The same tone is presented to both ears. The patient perceives the tone only in the ear where the sensation level is higher.

## The Stenger Test

The Stenger test is based on the Stenger effect. The purpose of the test is to identify functional or nonorganic hearing loss. It also can be used to estimate threshold in an individual who is demonstrating this type of hearing loss.

## When to Use the Stenger Test

The Stenger test can and should be used whenever there is a difference in air-conduction thresholds between ears of 20 dB or greater. It is best to perform the test immediately upon identifying a difference this large between ears.

## How to Administer the Stenger Test

The Stenger test can be administered using either pure tones or speech. Most audiometers have a function to administer the stimulus with the same phase, and this function must be utilized to deliver the stimulus. The intensity levels for the two ears should be set with the intensity of the "better" ear at 10 dB above threshold and the intensity of the "poorer" ear at 10 dB below the admitted threshold. The stimulus is then presented. No special instructions should be given to the patient. In short, the patient should not be aware that the examiner is performing this particular test. To avoid the need for giving further instruction, the Stenger test should be performed immediately upon identifying a difference of 20 dB or greater between ears. Conduct a pure-tone Stenger test during pure-tone testing. Likewise, conduct a speech Stenger test when you are testing using speech signals.

## Stenger Test Outcomes

If the patient responds to the tone or speech when the Stenger test is performed, then the test outcome is negative. The patient is demonstrating that the hearing loss is likely organic. If the patient fails to respond to the tone or speech, then the test outcome is positive. The patient is demonstrating that he or she likely has a functional or exaggerated hearing loss.

For example, imagine that you have a patient who demonstrates a unilateral hearing loss at 1000 Hz as shown in Figure 17–4.

Assume that the "truth" in this case is that the patient does have this loss. The first question is, "Can a Stenger test be performed in this situation?" The answer is "Yes," because there is a 50 dB difference between the thresholds. Next, we determine the intensity of the signal to be presented to each ear. For the right ear—the "better" ear—the signal is presented at 10 dB above threshold, 20 dB HL in this case. For the left ear—the "poorer" ear—the signal is presented at 10 dB below admitted threshold, 50 dB HL in this case, as shown in Figure 17–5.

The outcome of the test is shown in Figure 17–6. In this case, the patient has a sensation level of 10 dB in the right ear and −10 dB in the left ear. Due to the Stenger effect, the sound is perceived only in the ear with the higher sensation level. The patient perceives the sound in the right ear and responds appropriately, indicating that the sound was heard. This is a negative Stenger test result.

Now, using the same example, assume that the "truth" of the case is that the patient actually has a functional hearing loss in the left ear. The Stenger test is performed in the same manner, but the results, shown in Figure 17–7, are different. In this case, the patient has a sensation level of 10 dB in the right ear and 30 dB in the left ear. Due to the Stenger effect, the sound is heard only in the ear with the higher sensation level, the left ear. However, because the patient is unwilling to admit to hearing the tone in the left ear at such a low sensation level, the patient does not respond to the tone. This is a positive Stenger test result. It alerts the tester that the hearing loss is likely nonorganic or exaggerated.

## Threshold Estimation Using the Stenger Test

When a positive Stenger test outcome is found, the Stenger test can be used to estimate the

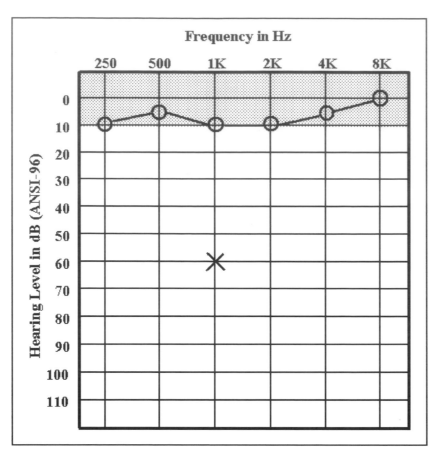

**FIGURE 17–4.** Audiogram showing a unilateral hearing loss at 1000 Hz.

Present to "better" ear at 10 dB above threshold

Present to "poorer" ear at 10 dB below threshold

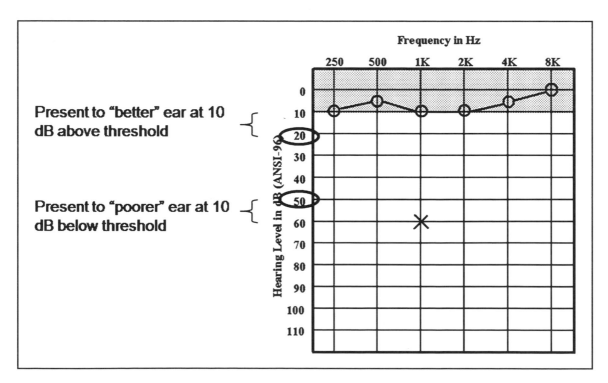

**FIGURE 17–5.** Audiogram demonstrating the presentation levels for the Stenger test based on reported thresholds.

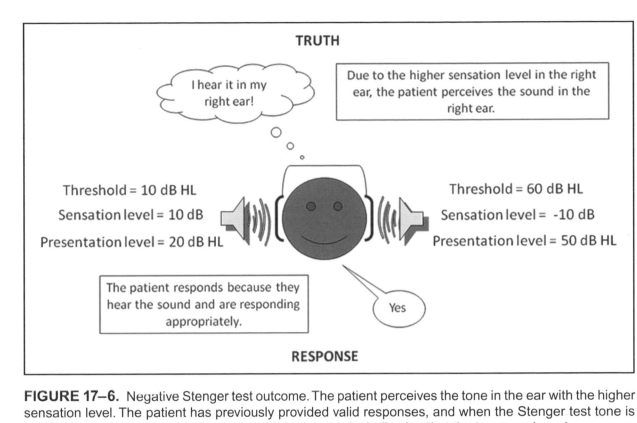

**FIGURE 17–6.** Negative Stenger test outcome. The patient perceives the tone in the ear with the higher sensation level. The patient has previously provided valid responses, and when the Stenger test tone is presented, the patient provides another valid response by indicating that the tone was heard.

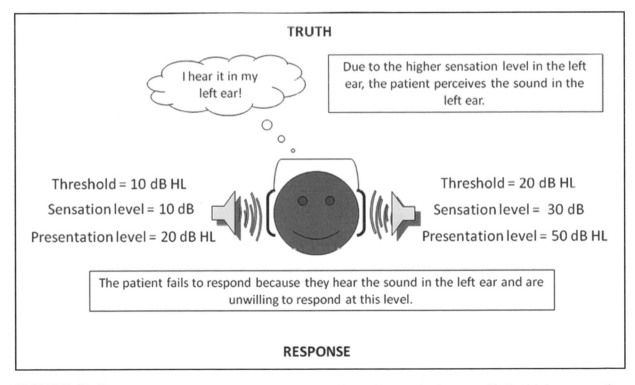

**FIGURE 17–7.** Positive Stenger test. The patient perceives the tone in the ear with the higher sensation level, the left ear. However, the patient has previously provided invalid responses, which would suggest that hearing in the left ear is actually poorer than it is. The patient cannot then admit that the tone was heard in the left ear. When the Stenger test tone is presented, the patient chooses not to respond to the tone.

patient's true threshold. To do this, the examiner decreases the presentation level of the sound in the "poorer" ear to 0 dB HL. The presentation level of the sound in the "good" ear remains at 10 dB SL. The stimulus is presented again simultaneously with the stimulus in the "good" ear, and the patient response is observed. When the patient responds, the presentation level to the "poorer" ear is raised by 5 dB and the stimulus is presented again. This process is repeated until the patient stops responding that the tone was heard.

When the patient responds, it means that the sensation level in the "good" ear is still better than the sensation level in the "poor" ear. If the patient fails to respond, it means that the sensation level in the "poor" ear has become greater than the sensation level in the "good" ear. Because the patient is not admitting to a sensation level this low, the patient stops responding. Based on experimental data, it is known that the intensity level at which the patient stops responding is

about 15 to 30 dB greater than the actual threshold. This allows estimation of the actual threshold of the ear in question.

Look at the previous example. Again, assume that the patient has a "true" threshold of 20 dB HL in the left ear but is responding to the tone at 60 dB HL. The clinician has performed the Stenger test and obtained a positive result. Now, the clinician wishes to estimate the actual threshold of the left ear. To accomplish this, the clinician lowers the intensity of the signal presented to the left ear to 0 dB HL. This lowers the sensation level of the left ear. The Stenger test is then repeated at this lower sensation level. The patient perceives the tone only in the right ear, and so responds to the tone, as shown in Figure 17–8.

This is repeated, raising the intensity level of the "poorer" left ear by 5 dB. Again, the sensation level of the right ear is greater than the left ear, and the patient continues to respond, as shown in Figure 17–9.

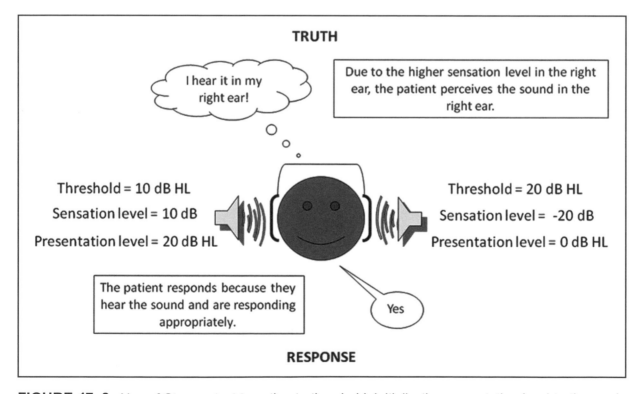

**FIGURE 17–8.** Use of Stenger test to estimate threshold. Initially, the presentation level to the ear in question is lowered to 0 dB HL. The patient truthfully only perceives the tone in the right ear, which has the higher sensation level. The patient accurately responds that the tone is perceived.

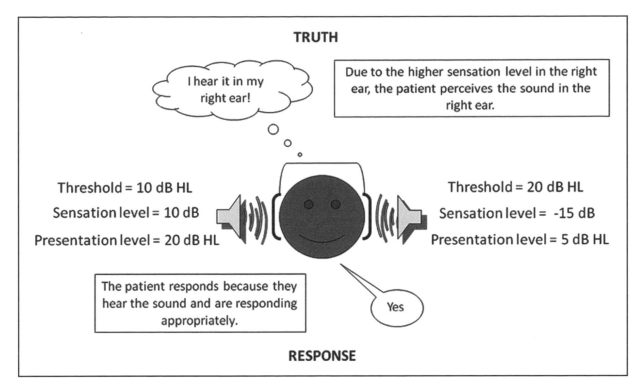

**FIGURE 17–9.** Use of Stenger test to estimate threshold. The presentation level to the ear in question is increased incrementally in 5 dB steps. Although the ear in question still has a sensation level below that of the other ear, the patient continues to perceive it in the other ear and will respond that the tone is perceived.

This is repeated in 5 dB steps until the patient fails to respond. For this patient, assume that this occurred at an intensity level of 40 dB HL in the left ear, as shown in Figure 17–10.

At this level, the patient began to perceive the sensation level in the left ear as being greater than in the right ear. However, the sensation level here is lower than the level at which the patient is will-ing to respond in the left ear. So the patient stops responding. We know then, that the patient's true threshold level is somewhat less than the intensity of the presentation level. From this information, it can be determined that the threshold is "better than" 40 dB HL, not 60 dB HL as the patient's previous responses would indicate.

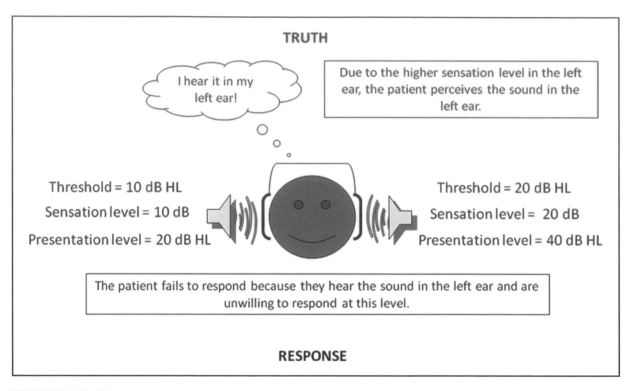

**FIGURE 17–10.** Use of Stenger test to estimate threshold. The presentation level to the ear in question continues to be increased until a sensation level is reached where the sound is actually perceived in the ear in question. At this point, the patient is unwilling to admit that it is heard in that ear, and so stops responding. This indicates that the patient's true threshold for the ear in question is at least less than or equal to the level at which the patient's affirmative responses ceased.

## OBSERVATION

1. Observe an experienced clinician administer the Stenger test to an individual with a unilateral hearing loss who provides accurate responses. *Note:* A unilateral hearing loss can be simulated in this case using a sound-attenuating foam insert plug in one ear.

2. Observe the clinician administer the Stenger test to a volunteer who exaggerates or feigns a hearing loss.

3. Observe the clinician utilize the Stenger test to estimate threshold in a volunteer who exaggerates or feigns a hearing loss.

## GUIDED PRACTICE

1. Obtain a pure-tone air-conduction audiogram for a volunteer with a unilateral hearing loss, or simulated unilateral hearing loss.

2. At a frequency where thresholds are shown to differ by 20 dB or greater, perform the Stenger test, using the listener's actual thresholds. Have the volunteer respond accurately.

3. Have the same volunteer feign a hearing loss and perform the Stenger test. *Note:* Have the volunteer "blind" you to conditions of accurate or feigned responses in steps 2 and 3 to demonstrate the effect.

4. Perform the Stenger test in the previous two conditions using speech instead of pure tones.

5. Have the volunteer feign a hearing loss and use the Stenger test to estimate the actual threshold of the listener.

## REFLECTION AND REVIEW

1. Describe the Stenger effect.

_____

_____

_____

_____

_____

2. What is the primary purpose of performing the Stenger test? What is a second possible use of the Stenger test?

_____

_____

3. Under what conditions can you perform a Stenger test?

_____

_____

4. Imagine that you are observing a hearing test. The audiologist finds a positive Stenger effect. The audiologist then reinstructs the patient saying, "Remember, please respond to the tones, even if they are very soft." Why might the audiologist choose to do this?

_____

_____

# ||| 18 |||

## Tuning Fork Tests

## INTRODUCTION

Tuning fork tests may be conducted to provide the audiologist with additional information regarding the patient's hearing loss. Although tuning fork tests may not be consistently used in every clinical situation, understanding the principles of these tests can help you better understand the auditory system as well as give you a range of tools to confirm your audiometric findings. This chapter addresses the procedures used for the most common tuning fork tests and how they relate to standard audiometric results.

## LEARNING OUTCOMES

- Be able to instruct patients to obtain valid tuning fork test results.
- Know how to interpret patient responses to tuning fork tests.
- Know how tuning fork test results relate to audiometric test results.

## REVIEW OF CONCEPTS

### Stimuli for Tuning Fork Tests

#### Use of a Tuning Fork

Using a tuning fork properly requires a bit of practice. When striking the fork, find a firm surface on which you will strike one of the tines, without damaging the surface itself. A rubber pad is recommended. Hold your arm slightly bent while firmly holding the base of the tuning of the fork. Tap just one of the tines about a third of the way down.

The choice of the frequency of the tuning fork is an important clinician consideration. Typically, tests that are used to examine conductive components of hearing loss are best tested with 512 Hz or lower-frequency tuning forks. Higher-frequency tuning forks will be useful when testing for high-frequency sensorineural hearing loss.

#### Use of a Bone Vibrator

Audiologists often use a bone vibrator to conduct an audiometric version of a tuning fork test. For example, during the Weber test, described shortly, the audiologist may place the bone vibrator in the center of the patient's forehead and conduct the testing with bone-conducted signals via the audiometer, rather than using a tuning fork. This has the advantage of presenting a calibrated signal.

## Patient Preparation

Prior to beginning testing, the audiologist must physically prepare the patient to be tested and must provide instructions to the patient so that the patient will provide valid behavioral responses.

The audiologist should request that the patient remove food, chewing gum, glasses, and head coverings. It is critical that the audiologist not inform the patient of the anticipated results of the different tuning fork tests.

Patients should be informed that at times, the tuning fork may be in contact with their head, and other times it will not. Regardless of the position of the tuning fork, the patient should respond as appropriate.

## Bing Test

The Bing test is based on the occlusion effect. In the case of normal hearing or sensorineural loss, the patient will perceive a bone-conducted signal as louder when the ear canal is closed versus open due to the occlusion effect. If there is a conductive loss where the breakdown in function causes an occlusion effect in either or both ears, no difference will be detected between open versus closed ear canal conditions because the disorder itself is already causing an occlusion effect.

To perform the test, instruct the patient that you will place the tuning fork behind her or his ear on the mastoid process. Tell the patient that after the tuning fork is on the mastoid, the patient should indicate whether he or she hears a tone. Then, the patient must tell you when the tone has "stopped" or is no longer perceived. When the patient indicates that he or she no longer perceives the tone, gently close the opening to the ear canal. Ask the patient to inform you if the sound

is heard again, in either ear. Alternatively, the base of the vibrating tuning fork can be placed on the patient's mastoid process while the clinician presses the tragus down to occlude the ear canal opening as the tines are vibrating. In this case, the patient makes the subjective indication whether the tone is "louder" when the ear canal is closed versus open.

A positive Bing test result occurs if the patient perceives the tone again or louder when the ear canal is occluded. In this case, it is likely that there is no conductive component because the patient is now perceiving the tone due to the enhancement of the signal caused by the occlusion effect that you created by closure of the ear canal. A negative Bing test result occurs if the patient does not perceive the tone again, or perceives no difference, with the ear canal occluded. In this case, there is likely a conductive hearing loss because the disordered middle ear system was already resulting in an occlusion effect prior to manual occlusion of the ear canal.

## Rinne Test

The Rinne test is useful for differentiating between normal hearing or sensorineural loss and conductive hearing loss. In patients with normal middle ear function and normal hearing sensitivity or sensorineural hearing loss, the patient will perceive a bone-conducted signal as softer than the same air-conducted signal from the tuning fork. This is because air conduction is more efficient than bone conduction. In the case of a conductive hearing loss, the patient will perceive the bone-conducted signal as louder because the pathology causing the hearing loss has created a less efficient system for transmission of the air-conducted signal.

To perform the test, strike a low-frequency tuning fork and place it about 2 inches from the ear canal of the patient. Ask the patient if the tone is perceived by instructing the patient to, "Raise your hand as long as you hear the tone." When the patient's hand is lowered, place the base of the tuning fork on the mastoid process of the patient. Ask the patient, "Do you hear the tone again?" If the tone returns, the test is considered a negative

Rinne result, indicating a conductive component. If the tone is no longer present, the test is considered a positive Rinne result. This is consistent with the absence of a conductive hearing loss. Another method for performing this test is to hold the tuning fork near the ear canal for a given period of time and then move the fork to the mastoid process. In this case, the patient should respond by indicating in which case the tone was louder. If the tone is reported as louder while the tuning fork is held near the ear canal, this is a positive Rinne because the signal should be more efficiently perceived via air conduction. This condition is consistent with either normal hearing sensitivity or a sensorineural hearing loss. If the tone is reported as louder while the tuning fork is placed on the mastoid, this is a negative Rinne result because the occlusion effect caused by the pathology is causing the signal to be perceived more efficiently via bone conduction. *Note*: A challenge with the Rinne test is that if the contralateral ear is not masked, it will be difficult for the clinician to determine exactly which ear is responding in the bone conduction condition.

## Schwabach Test

The Schwabach test is conducted to determine the presence of hearing loss by bone conduction. It is crucial for the person conducting the test to have thresholds at audiometric zero for the test results to be valid, thereby making this particular tuning fork test one of the least likely to be clinically useful. The frequency of the tuning fork used for this test is chosen based on the frequency at which hearing loss is suspected. For this test, the tuning fork is struck and placed on the mastoid of the patient. The patient informs the clinician when the tone is no longer heard. The clinician then places the fork on his or her own mastoid process to determine the presence of the tone. If the tone is still present, the clinician determines how long (in seconds) he or she perceives the tone beyond that of the patient. To correlate the findings of this test with the pure-tone audiogram, the clinician must know the decay rate of the tuning fork in use. For instance, if the tone decays at a rate of 5 dB per

second and the clinician has perceived the tone for 6 seconds longer than the patient, it can be determined that the patient has a 30 dB HL hearing loss, assuming that the audiometric thresholds for the clinician are at 0 dB HL.

To perform this test, instruct the patient that you will place the base of the tuning fork on the patient's mastoid process. Say, "Raise your hand for as long as you hear the tone." Now, strike the fork and place the base on the patient's mastoid. As soon as the patient indicates that the tone is no longer audible, place the fork next on your own mastoid and begin timing in seconds until the tone is no longer audible to you.

There are three basic outcomes to the test, assuming that the examiner has normal hearing. First, the patient could have normal hearing by bone conduction. Second, the patient could hear the tone longer than the examiner (or possibly for the same amount of time), indicating a conductive hearing loss. Finally, the patient could have a sensorineural hearing loss if he or she hears the tone for a shorter time period than the examiner. The Schwabach test is rarely used to identify hearing loss due to the wide availability of clinical audiometers. Results from this test should be interpreted with caution due to the many variables that can impact the results.

## Weber Test

The Weber test is performed to determine the presence of a conductive component in the case of unilateral hearing loss. This test is based on both the occlusion effect and the Stenger effect. For this test, a low-frequency tuning fork is struck, and the base is placed on the forehead or frontal sinuses. The patient is instructed to tell the examiner in which ear the tone is heard. It is important to instruct the patient that he or she might hear the tone in the better ear, the worse ear, or possibly somewhere else in the head.

For patients who have a conductive hearing loss in one ear, an occlusion effect is created in that ear, causing a higher sensation level. When the tuning fork is placed onto the forehead, a tone of the same intensity and phase is presented to both ears simultaneously. Due to the Stenger effect, the patient hears the tone only in the ear with the higher sensation level. Because the occlusion effect creates a higher sensation level, the patient reports hearing the sound in the ear with the conductive hearing loss.

For patients who have a sensorineural hearing loss in one ear, there is no occlusion effect. The patient has a higher sensation level in the opposite ear and will report hearing the sound in that ear,

again due to the Stenger effect. Another way to say this is that the tone will localize to the ear with the conductive component or to the ear with the better sensorineural reserve. In some cases, patients are unable to differentiate in which ear the sound was heard, and the test outcome is equivocal.

Finally, patients with normal hearing, as well as some with bilateral sensorineural hearing loss, may report hearing the tone in both ears or "all over" the head.

## OBSERVATION

1. Observe an experienced clinician conduct a Bing test.

2. Examine how the results of the Bing tuning fork test relate to the patient's audiogram near the frequency tested.

3. Observe the clinician conduct a Rinne test.

4. Examine how the results of the Rinne tuning fork test relate to the patient's audiogram near the frequency tested.

5. Observe the clinician conduct a Schwabach test.

6. Examine how the results of the Schwabach tuning fork test relate to the patient's audiogram near the frequency tested.

7. Observe the clinician conduct a Weber test.

8. Examine how the results of the Weber tuning fork test relate to the patient's audiogram near the frequency tested.

## GUIDED PRACTICE

1. Instruct a patient to respond for the Bing test.

2. Obtain results of the Bing test for a patient.

3. Instruct a patient to respond for the Rinne test.

4. Obtain results of the Rinne test for a patient.

5. Place a foam plug in the ear of the volunteer and repeat the Rinne test.

6. Instruct a patient to respond for the Schwabach test.

7. Obtain results of the Schwabach test for a patient.

8. Place a foam plug in the ear of the volunteer and repeat the Schwabach test.

9. Place a foam plug in the ear of a volunteer and instruct the patient to respond for the Weber test.

10. Obtain results of the Weber test for a patient.

## REFLECTION AND REVIEW

1. Describe in detail the instructions you would provide to a patient on whom you are about to perform the Bing test.

_____

_____

_____

_____

_____

2. Describe in detail the instructions you would provide to a patient on whom you are about to perform the Rinne test.

_____

_____

_____

3. Describe in detail the instructions you would provide to a patient on whom you are about to perform the Schwabach test.

_____

_____

_____

_____

_____

4. Describe in detail the instructions you would provide to a patient on whom you are about to perform the Weber test.

_____

_____

_____

_____

5. What frequency tuning forks are used for different tuning fork tests? How do the different frequency forks impact your results?

_____

_____

_____

_____

6. Think of all of the different tests possible in the case of a patient with unilateral conductive hearing loss. What would you expect the results to be? What about in the case of a bilateral conductive loss? Finally, consider the patient with bilateral symmetric sensorineural hearing loss.

_____

_____

_____

_____

7. What are the benefits of tuning fork tests as whole? What are the limitations?

_____

_____

_____

_____

8. Examine the audiogram in Figure 18–1. Assume that you performed a Weber test. Which ear should the sound localize to in the Weber test if audiometric results are valid?

_____

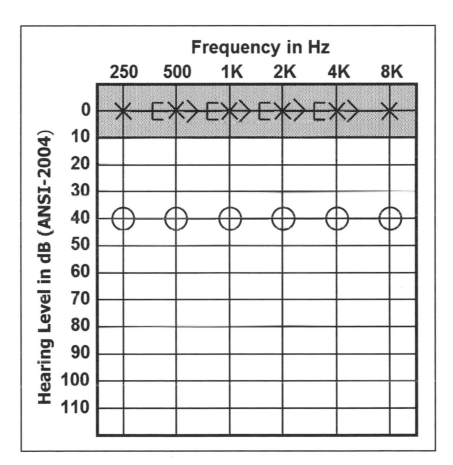

**FIGURE 18–1.** Audiogram demonstrating unilateral conductive hearing loss.

9. Examine the audiogram in Figure 18–2. Which tuning fork tests could help to confirm that the hearing loss is sensorineural in nature?

_____

_____

_____

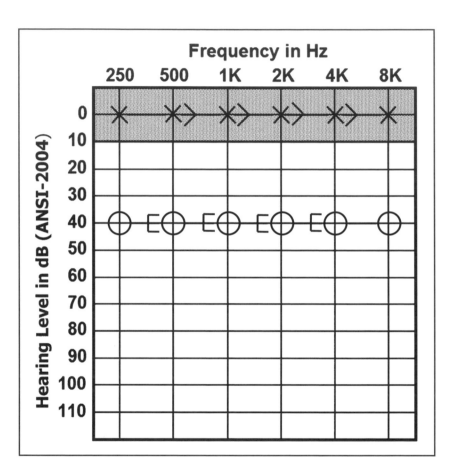

**FIGURE 18–2.** Audiogram demonstrating unilateral sensorineural hearing loss.

# ║║║ 19 ║║║

## Otoacoustic Emissions

### INTRODUCTION

Otoacoustic emissions (OAEs) are vibrations generated as by-products of the mechanical action of the outer hair cells of the cochlea. These pressure waves travel "backward" through the structures of the ear, vibrate the tympanic membrane, and generate very low-intensity sounds that can be measured in the ear canal. Measurement of OAEs provides an objective means of determining the functionality of outer hair cells.

The outer hair cells are responsible for hearing the softest sounds. Their presence or absence can be valuable clinically for a number of reasons. These include, but are not limited to, understanding function of hearing in children and difficult-to-test populations, identifying functional or exaggerated hearing loss, monitoring hearing of those taking ototoxic medications, and in some cases, distinguishing between cochlear and retro-cochlear pathology.

This chapter covers basic principles of OAE generation and recording. The reader is encouraged to pursue an in-depth study of these topics in other texts (such as that by Dhar & Hall, 2012).

### LEARNING OUTCOMES

- Understand the types of OAEs that can be measured.
- Know the patient behaviors required for testing of OAEs.
- Know how to obtain appropriate OAE recordings.

### REVIEW OF CONCEPTS

#### What Are Otoacoustic Emissions?

Otoacoustic emissions are vibrations generated by the mechanical processes of the outer hair cells of the cochlea. These pressure waves are transmitted through the structures of the inner, middle, and outer ear in the opposite direction to the forward transmission of sound vibrations that generated them.

During forward transmission of sound vibration, the basilar membrane of the cochlea is displaced by the forward "traveling wave." In a healthy ear, at the area of maximal displacement of the basilar membrane, the outer hair cells contract to bring the tectorial membrane closer to the inner hair cells. This changes the movement of fluid in the cochlea, increasing the likelihood of inner hair cell stimulation to generate an action potential. The effect of this outer hair cell activity is to elicit stimulation at a lower intensity level and at a more finely tuned frequency than would otherwise occur.

The contraction of the outer hair cells also creates movement of the cochlear fluids, and this motion is propagated toward the round and oval windows. When these pressure waves reach the oval window, the ossicles are set into motion, which in turn creates motion of the tympanic membrane. The tympanic membrane movement acts as a loudspeaker, creating pressure waves in the ear canal, which result in sound. This sound is called an *otoacoustic emission*.

## How Are Otoacoustic Emissions Related to Auditory Disorder?

Otoacoustic emissions reflect the integrity of outer hair cell function. Ears that are functioning normally will produce measureable OAEs.

Most sensorineural hearing loss begins with the loss of outer hair cell function. These cells seem particularly susceptible to noise, toxins, and the aging process. So patients with sensorineural hearing loss will most often have a loss of outer hair cells, resulting in a loss of OAEs. As a general rule, when a sensorineural hearing loss reaches 20 dB, the probability of measuring OAEs becomes quite low and falls off precipitously as hearing loss increases.

Less commonly, sensorineural hearing loss is caused by problems beyond the outer hair cells. In such cases, the patient will present with a sensorineural hearing loss but with preserved OAEs. In these rare cases the loss is caused by inner hair cell loss, a disorder of the VIIIth nerve, or a disorder of the communication between inner hair cells and VIIIth nerve fibers.

Conductive hearing loss, caused by outer and middle ear disorder has a variable effect on OAEs. For example, in more involved cases of middle ear disorder, the OAE will occur in the cochlea but will not be transmitted effectively back through the middle ear, and the OAEs will not be measureable. In milder cases, the OAEs may be of sufficient intensity to be recorded in the ear canal.

## Types of OAEs

OAEs can occur spontaneously. In a healthy ear they are also generated in response to the occurrence of sounds that are heard by the patient. In order to make use of the OAEs that occur in the ear canal to understand the health of outer hair cell function in the cochlea, it is helpful to evoke their presence so that they can be systematically measured. OAEs can be evoked by presentation of calibrated sound stimuli into the ear canal. When OAEs occur as a function of stimulation, they are known as *evoked otoacoustic emissions* (EOAEs).

There are several ways in which OAEs can be evoked and measured. The EOAEs that are in widespread clinical use are *transient evoked otoacoustic emissions* (TEOAEs) and *distortion product evoked otoacoustic emissions* (DPOAEs).

TEOAEs are evoked with a transient stimulus (i.e., a click). The click stimulus is broad spectrum in nature, allowing for the majority of the basilar membrane to be stimulated nearly simultaneously. Thus, information about the outer hair cell function along much of the basilar membrane is elicited with each stimulus.

DPOAEs are evoked using two tones of fixed frequency and intensity. When tones have a particular frequency ratio to one another, distortions are created by the active mechanism of the cochlea. The mechanics of the basilar membrane movement cause the stimulation of outer hair cells at frequencies other than the stimulating tones that are mathematically related to the frequencies of the stimulating tones. Vibrations that occur due to outer hair cell function at these additional frequencies are known as distortion product otoacoustic emissions. When DPOAEs are measured in the ear canal, they provide information about the health of the outer hair cells at the frequencies of the stimulation tones. There are numerous DPOAEs that are generated in response to stimulation by two tones of a particular frequency ratio.

For general clinical use, two tones are presented known as f1 and f2, with f1 being the lower-frequency tone and f2 being the higher frequency of the two tones. It has been empirically determined that the optimal frequency ratio of these stimulus tones is approximately 1.2. The stimulus tones also have empirically determined intensity levels, known as L1 and L2 (corresponding to the respective frequencies of f1 and f2). The most commonly used intensities of these two tones for general clinical use are 65 dB SPL for L1 (f1) and 55 dB SPL for L2 (f2). The distortion product that is most commonly used is known as the *cubic difference distortion product*. The formula for its frequency is 2f1 − f2.

## Equipment

Equipment used for OAE testing generally comes in two forms: screening and diagnostic. Screening equipment generally does not allow for manipulation of testing parameters and, in some cases, may not provide a result beyond "presence" or "absence" of emissions. Diagnostic equipment generally allows for multiple types of emissions to be measured, allows for manipulation of testing parameters, and provides numeric results for interpretation by the clinician.

OAE testing equipment consists of a computer that is used to generate a calibrated acoustic signal. The digital signal is transmitted via a cord that connects to a probe where the acoustic signal is generated. The probe has a loudspeaker for delivery of the test signal and a highly sensitive microphone to measure the sounds occurring in the ear canal.

The signals that occur in the ear canal include the test stimuli, ambient and physiologic noise, and all of the evoked OAEs that occur in response to the test stimuli. Measurement of the test stimuli is helpful to ensure that the signal presented into the ear canal is of the desired frequency and intensity. These signals are measured, and, on diagnostic equipment, they can be inspected to ensure that the measurement was made using appropriate stimuli.

There is an additional large amount of extraneous sound in the ear canal from environmental and physiologic sources that is random relative to the time-locked evoked otoacoustic emission. In order to reduce the amount of unwanted noise relative to the OAE of interest, a signal averaging system is employed. The test stimuli are presented numerous times and the responses recorded each time. The number of times that test stimuli are presented depends on the parameters set by the clinician and the "stopping rules" that are criteria that include intensity level of the noise floor, intensity level of OAEs, differences between these values, and duration of the test time. These responses are averaged, thereby reducing sounds emanating from random extraneous sources. In contrast, the signal of interest, which is time locked to the presentation of the stimuli, begins to emerge from the background noise. In addition, signals that include noise that exceeds a particular intensity level are rejected to prevent contamination of the response.

## TEOAE Testing Parameters

Test stimuli parameters for TEOAEs are typically fixed on most clinical equipment and offer very few parameters that can be adjusted. In some cases, the number of samples obtained, stopping criteria, rejection threshold, and stimulus intensity can be adjusted as needed.

## DPOAE Testing Parameters

There are several parameters that can often be adjusted when performing DPOAE testing. The choice of parameters used will depend on the purpose of DPOAE testing and the conditions under which the test is occurring. One such parameter is the range of frequencies tested. DPOAEs can be elicited across a range of frequencies, and the reason for testing can provide rationale for the range of frequencies tested. For example, in the case of a patient who is being tested to assess the effects of ototoxic medications on the auditory system, very high-frequency DPOAE evaluation may be used to understand effects of ototoxic medications early in the course of treatment. In the case of a young child who is having a cross-check of behavioral hearing responses, the frequency range tested may be limited to a more standard audiometric range.

Another variable that may be manipulated with some equipment is the number of test points per octave that are assessed. This measure dictates how fine-tuned the measurements are within an octave band. The more measurements that are made within an octave band, the more frequency-specific information can be obtained. As with the range of frequencies, the choice of the number of test points per octave is made depending on the purposes of testing. In some cases, a highly precise frequency location of dysfunction may provide useful information for diagnosis or treatment.

As described previously, the frequency and intensity ratios most typically used for eliciting DPOAEs in clinical practice are chosen to provide the most robust cubic difference distortion product across the frequencies most typically tested. However, there may be specific circumstances in which the frequency or intensity ratio should be altered, and some equipment provides opportunity to adjust these parameters.

## Environmental and Patient Conditions

The transmission of vibrations "backward" through the structures of the cochlea and middle ear is far less efficient than "forward" transmission through these structures. Because of this, the OAEs recorded in the ear canal are very low in intensity. The measurement of such low-intensity sounds requires that the environment in which OAEs are measured be very quiet. A sound booth is the ideal location for such measurements to occur, but OAEs can be measured elsewhere, as long as the environment is made as quiet as possible.

In addition to a quiet environment, a quiet patient is essential to the process of effectively recording OAEs. This can typically be achieved by instructing a compliant adult or older child that they will be hearing sounds and that their job is to sit as still and quiet as possible throughout the testing. In infants, the testing is best carried out in natural sleep but can be accomplished as long as the infant is awake but quiet. An infant who has been fed and is comfortable is typically necessary for this. A pacifier or soother is often helpful for calming awake infants. For young children, the clinician must ensure that the child does not purposefully or inadvertently pull the earphone out of the ear. The child must also be kept as still and calm as possible. The parent or caregiver's assistance is typically necessary, and most young children do well sitting on the lap of this person. Any number of techniques may be employed to distract the child and maintain the child's quiet attention, including showing the child a picture book, allowing the child to watch an animation with no sound, having the child hold quiet toys, and so on.

*Clinical Note*: You are likely to encounter cases in clinical practice where OAEs cannot be recorded due to respiratory illness in patients. Labored and wheezing breathing cause excessive noise in the ear canal, and these physiologic sounds make recording OAEs impossible in some cases.

*Clinical Note:* Physiologic noises are typically low frequency, and therefore it is much more difficult to record low-frequency OAEs.

An otoscopic examination should be conducted prior to patient testing. Cerumen, drainage, or other debris in the ear canal can impede the transmission of sound in the ear canal and should be removed prior to testing. In addition, otoscopic examination may reveal indications of middle ear disorder, such as observable fluid behind the tympanic membrane or a bulging tympanic membrane. Findings on tympanometry may also be used to verify the health of the middle ear. Fluid in the middle ear space or other middle ear dysfunction will attenuate the transmission of sound to the ear canal, and knowledge of the presence of these factors is helpful when interpreting results.

## Recording OAEs

Once the equipment is set and the patient prepared, actually recording OAEs is simply a matter of pressing "start" on the computer. The stimuli will be presented and measurements made automatically by the equipment. The job of the clinician during this time is to observe the calibration measures to ensure that the recording is being conducted properly and to maintain the optimal environmental conditions (quiet) and patient behaviors (still and quiet) for recording the sounds. In compliant adults this is generally a simple task. In infants and young children and difficult-to-test patients, this may require much skill on the part of the audiologist.

## Interpretation of OAE recordings

TEOAE recordings are commonly displayed using a table of values, a graphical display of two bins of averaged waveforms (intensity of the emission as a function of time) elicited by the stimulus, and a graphical display of the intensity of the sound measured in the ear canal as a function of frequency. An example of this output can be seen in Figure 19–1.

Two types of outcomes can be evaluated with TEOAEs. An overall assessment of the presence of an OAE response can be determined, or the response can be divided into frequency regions to be more discretely evaluated.

In addition, there are two values that can be used to determine the presence or absence of a TEOAE response. One value of importance is the reproducibility of the response. Each consecutive recording of the response is stored in one of two "bins." The responses are then compared to determine the percentage that is the same, or reproducibility, between the two responses. In addition, the levels of the TEOAE and the noise floor levels are used to determine whether the TEOAE of interest is present. The TEOAE must be sufficiently intense to be considered a potential TEOAE and must be sufficiently higher than the noise floor to be considered present and not just a signal occurring randomly in the background noise. The particular levels that allow a clinician to make that judgment depend on the normative data for the equipment and clinical population of interest.

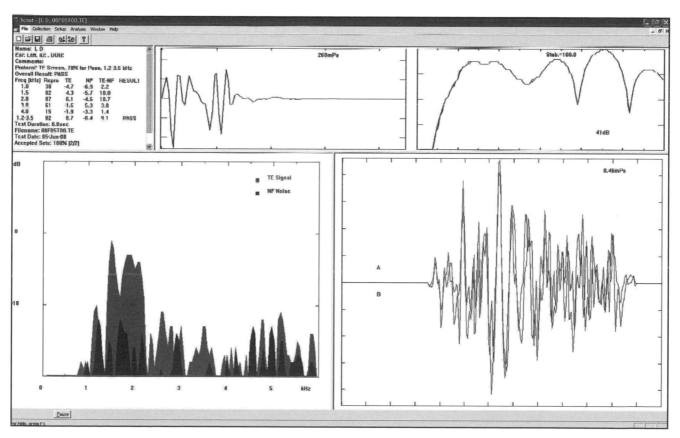

**FIGURE 19–1.** Data collection and analysis screen for a TEOAE system. (Image courtesy of Natus Medical Incorporated.)

A very rough guideline would be a difference between the DPOAE and the noise floor of 6 dB.

DPOAE recordings are commonly displayed using a table of values and a DP-gram, which is a graphical display of the intensity of the sound measured in the ear canal as a function of frequency. An example of this output can be seen in Figure 19–2. The DP-gram typically includes the intensity of f1, the intensity of f2, the intensity of the frequency of the cubic difference distortion product, and the intensity of predetermined frequencies present in the recording that are used to estimate the noise floor. The intensities of f1 and f2 are used to determine whether the signals intended to evoke the DPOAE were delivered at the correct frequency and intensities. The levels of the DPOAE and the noise floor levels are used to determine whether the DPOAE of interest is present. The DPOAE must be sufficiently intense to be considered a potential DPOAE and must be sufficiently higher than the noise floor to be considered to be present and not just a signal occurring randomly in the background noise. The particular levels that allow a clinician to make that judgment depend on the normative data for the equipment and clinical population of interest. A very rough guideline would be a difference between the DPOAE and the noise floor of 6 dB.

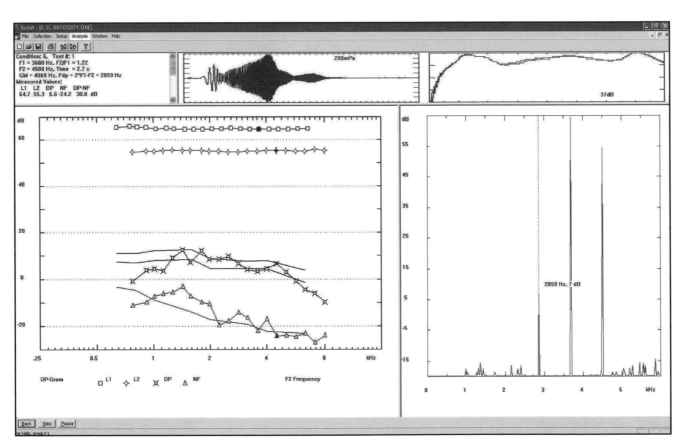

**FIGURE 19–2.** Data collection and analysis screen for a DPOAE system. (Image courtesy of Natus Medical Incorporated.)

## OBSERVATION

1. Observe an experienced clinician selecting testing parameters for TEOAE testing.

2. Observe an experienced clinician prepare a patient for and provide instructions for TEOAE testing.

3. Observe an experienced clinician elicit TEOAE measures for a patient.

4. Observe an experienced clinician selecting testing parameters for DPOAE testing.

5. Observe an experienced clinician prepare a patient for and provide instructions for DPOAE testing.

6. Observe an experienced clinician elicit DPOAE measures for a patient.

## GUIDED PRACTICE

1. Record TEOAEs for a classmate, friend, or family member.

2. Record DPOAEs for a classmate, friend, or family member.

3. Conduct an audiometric evaluation on the same individual and compare the behavioral audiometric results to the OAE measures.

4. Manipulate parameters of both tests and see how these changes impact results.

## REFLECTION AND REVIEW

1. What is the likely outcome of recording OAEs in an environment with substantial background noise?

_____

_____

_____

2. How would middle ear dysfunction impact the ability to record OAEs? Why?

_____

_____

_____

3. If a patient has present OAEs, but there are known indications of substantial hearing loss and poor word recognition, where would be the likely site of auditory dysfunction (outer ear, middle ear, cochlea, and/or VIIIth nerve or brainstem)?

_____

4. How would patient movement during testing impact the ability to record OAEs? Why?

_____

_____

_____

5. Why are low-frequency sounds seldom tested using OAEs?

_____

_____

6. What are the parameters (frequency and intensity ratios) of the stimuli used for DPOAE testing? Why are these particular parameters so frequently used?

_____

_____

_____

7. Explain the purpose of outer hair cell function.

_____

_____

_____

_____

8. How might OAEs be used in the identification of feigned or exaggerated hearing loss?

_____

_____

9. How might OAEs be used for monitoring of hearing in cases of administration of ototoxic medications?

_____

_____

# ||| 20 |||

## Interpreting Test Results

The most important function that you, as the audiologist, will perform during the audiologic assessment is to provide an interpretation of the function of the auditory system, using the data collected.

### LEARNING OUTCOMES

- Know the questions that should be answered for the purposes of the audiologic assessment.
- Begin to be able to analyze data to determine the function of the auditory system.

### REVIEW OF CONCEPTS

The importance of the "first question"—the reason for an audiologic evaluation to occur—was discussed in Chapter 2. The main outcome of interpretation of the audiologic results should be to provide information to support the goal(s) of the patient and the referring physician.

There are additional questions that the audiologic test outcomes should provide answers to, with the focus differing depending on the purpose for the evaluation. One issue that must be determined regardless of the rationale for testing is the validity of testing outcomes. Test validity can be assessed in a number of ways, and before drawing conclusions about the function of the auditory system, the audiologist must determine whether the testing outcomes are an accurate reflection of function.

In general, there are four areas of concern for the clinician regarding function of the auditory system: middle ear function, hearing sensitivity, retrocochlear function, and communication function. The measures collected during the audiologic exam generally contribute to understanding more than one of these areas of function and provide little useful information when considered in isolation. The role of the clinician is to incorporate all aspects of the audiologic evaluation to understand each area of audiologic function.

### Middle Ear Function

A major area of concern for many patients and physicians is the function of the middle ear system. Tympanometric and acoustic reflex immittance results, audiometric thresholds, otoacoustic emissions, and word recognition testing all add information to understanding the function of the middle ear system.

In general, middle ear dysfunction is characterized by abnormal tympanometric results, abnormal acoustic reflex immittance results, and air-bone gaps on the audiogram consistent with conductive hearing loss. In addition, in most cases of middle ear disorder otoacoustic emission responses cannot be recorded due to the attenuation of the backward transmission of sound. Therefore they will be "absent." Furthermore, word recognition testing results are typically better in the case of conductive hearing loss than they would be in the case of sensorineural hearing loss.

In some cases of middle ear dysfunction, such as otosclerosis, tympanometric results may appear normal, but acoustic reflex results will be abnormal with a corresponding conductive hearing loss indicated by air-bone gaps on the audiogram.

In the case of third-window syndromes, where there is no middle ear disorder, it is typical to find air-bone gaps on the audiogram, with normal typanometric and acoustic reflex immittance results, and otoacoustic emissions and word recognition results consistent with the degree of air-conduction hearing thresholds.

## Hearing Sensitivity

The presence or absence of hearing loss is a central aspect of the interpretation of the audiologic evaluation. When hearing loss is present, the hearing loss should be quantified according to the type, degree, and configuration of the hearing loss. The type of hearing loss is typically characterized as conductive, sensorineural, or mixed. The presence or absence of significant air-bone gaps on the audiogram provide information required to understand the type of hearing loss. In the case of significant air-bone gaps the hearing loss is typically described as conductive. In the case of absence of significant air-bone gaps the hearing loss is typically described as sensorineural. In the case of presence of air-bone gaps and elevated bone-conduction thresholds, the hearing loss is typically described as mixed.

*Clinical Note:* In some cases, such as third-window syndromes with the presence of air-bone gaps, the hearing loss is not "conductive" in the sense that it is typically used in describing results. In such cases it may be most useful to the referring provider when interpreting results to refer to the "air-bone gap" rather than to use the term "conductive."

The degree of hearing loss should be described using common terminology (mild, severe, etc.). The configuration of the hearing loss should also be described using common terminology (high-frequency, low-frequency, flat, etc).

## Retrocochlear Function

When a sensorineural hearing loss is identified it is important to obtain information to help distinguish as much as possible between a primarily sensory (cochlear) hearing loss and a primarily neural hearing loss. In cases of sensorineural hearing loss of primarily cochlear origin, the acoustic reflex thresholds, OAE results, and word recognition scores should be consistent with the degree of hearing sensitivity. In cases where the hearing loss is of strictly neural origin, acoustic reflex thresholds may be absent at hearing sensitivity levels where they would typically be present. In contrast OAE results may be present at hearing sensitivity levels where they would typically be absent. Word recognition results may be poorer than expected based on audiometric thresholds or when there is rollover of word recognition score performance at high intensities. When there is significant asymmetry between ears with regard to pure-tone thresholds or word recognition scores, concern is raised regarding retrocochlear pathology.

## Communication Function

The degree of hearing sensitivity loss as well as speech audiometric outcomes help to provide an understanding of the patient's communication function. Coupled with the patient's history, these outcomes should be considered to begin to determine the need for audiologic intervention, whether by amplification or other means.

# GUIDED PRACTICE

Review the audiometric case studies presented in Figures 20–1 through 20–6 and answer the following questions.

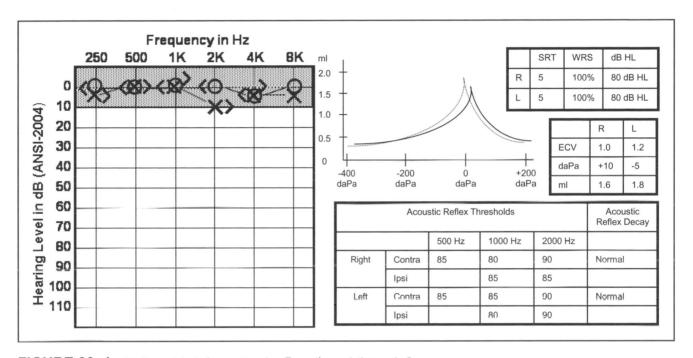

**FIGURE 20–1.** Audiometric information for Questions 1 through 3.

1. Is middle ear function normal?

_____

2. Is hearing loss present?

_____

3. Are test results in agreement?

_____

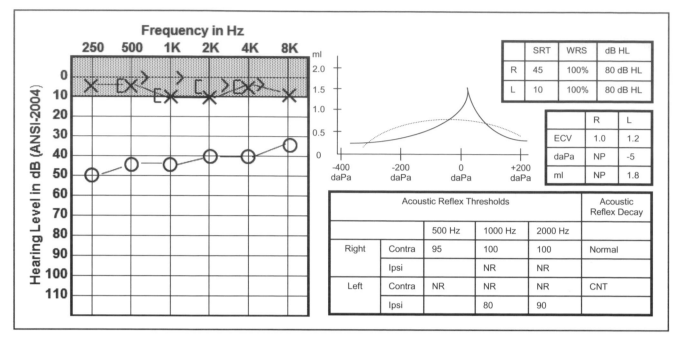

**FIGURE 20–2.** Audiometric information for Questions 4 through 9.

4. For the left ear, is middle ear function normal? Explain.

_____

5. For the right ear, is middle ear function normal? Explain.

_____

6. For the left ear, is hearing loss present? If so, describe the type, degree, and configuration of the hearing loss.

_____

7. For the right ear, is hearing loss present? If so, describe the type, degree, and configuration of the hearing loss.

_____

8. Are test results in agreement?

_____

9. What types of pathology might cause this pattern of audiologic function?

_____

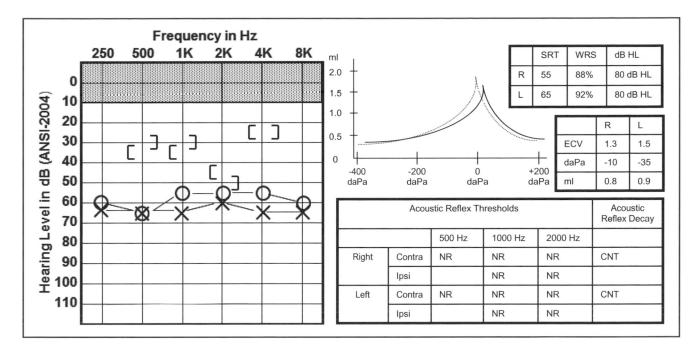

**FIGURE 20–3.** Audiometric information for Questions 10 through 15.

10. For the left ear, is middle ear function normal? Explain.

_____

11. For the right ear, is middle ear function normal? Explain.

_____

12. For the left ear, is hearing loss present? If so, describe the type, degree, and configuration of the hearing loss.

_____

13. For the right ear, is hearing loss present? If so, describe the type, degree, and configuration of the hearing loss.

_____

14. Are test results in agreement?

_____

15. What type of pathology might cause this pattern of audiologic function?

_____

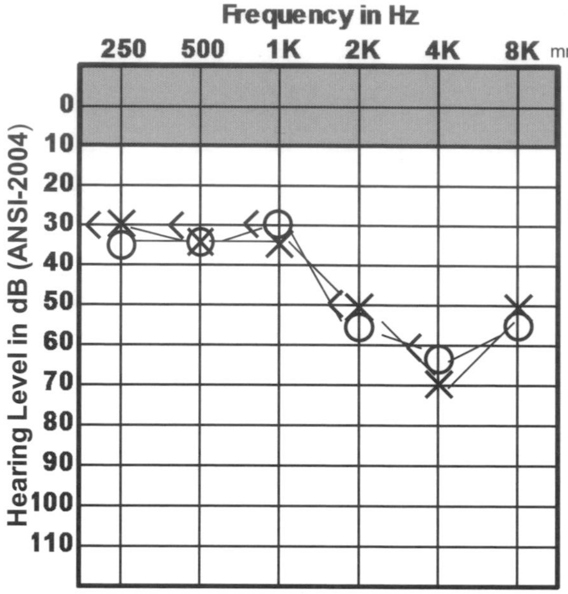


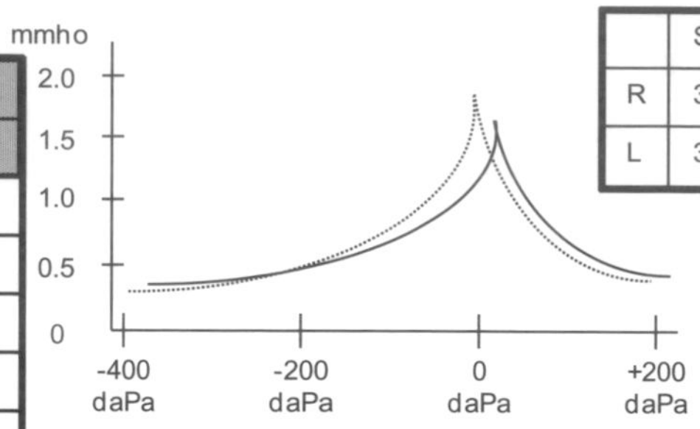


| | SRT | WRS | dB HL |
|---|---|---|---|
| R | 30 | 84% | 80 dB HL |
| L | 30 | 80% | 80 dB HL |

| | R | L |
|---|---|---|
| ECV | 1.0 | 1.2 |
| daPa | +10 | -5 |
| MI | 1.6 | 1.8 |

| Acoustic Reflex Thresholds | | | | | Acoustic Reflex Decay |
|---|---|---|---|---|---|
| | | 500 Hz | 1000 Hz | 2000 Hz | |
| Right | Contra | 90 | 90 | 100 | Normal |
| | Ipsi | | 95 | 100 | |
| Left | Contra | 95 | 90 | 105 | Normal |
| | Ipsi | | 95 | 105 | |

**FIGURE 20–4.** Audiometric information for Questions 16 through 21.

16. For the left ear, is middle ear function normal? Explain.

_______________

17. For the right ear, is middle ear function normal? Explain.

_______________

18. For the left ear, is hearing loss present? If so, describe the type, degree, and configuration of the hearing loss.

_______________

19. For the right ear, is hearing loss present? If so, describe the type, degree, and configuration of the hearing loss.

_______________

20. Are test results in agreement?

_______________

21. What type of pathology might cause this pattern of audiologic function?

_______________

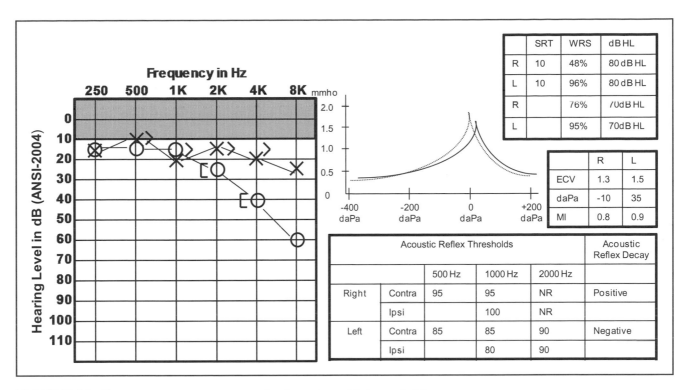

**FIGURE 20–5.** Audiometric information for Questions 22 through 30.

22. For the left ear, is middle ear function normal? Explain.

_____

23. For the right ear, is middle ear function normal? Explain.

_____

24. For the left ear, is hearing loss present? If so, describe the type, degree, and configuration of the hearing loss.

_____

25. For the right ear, is hearing loss present? If so, describe the type, degree, and configuration of the hearing loss.

_____

26. Are test results in agreement?

_____

27. Describe word recognition performance. What phenomenon is occurring for the right ear?

_____

_____

28. Describe acoustic reflex threshold patterns.

_____

_____

29. Describe acoustic reflex decay results.

_____

_____

30. What type of pathology might cause this pattern of audiologic function? Describe the overall pattern of results that would lead you to this concern.

_____

_____

_____

_____

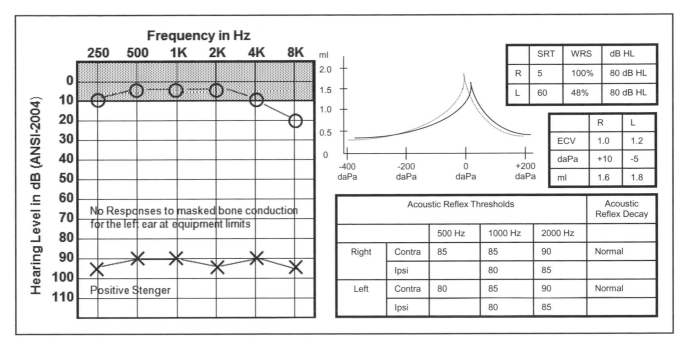

**FIGURE 20–6.** Audiometric information for Questions 31 through 36.

31. For the left ear, is middle ear function normal? Explain.

_____

32. For the right ear, is middle ear function normal? Explain.

_____

33. For the left ear, is hearing loss present? If so, describe the type, degree, and configuration of the hearing loss.

_____

34. For the right ear, is hearing loss present? If so, describe the type, degree, and configuration of the hearing loss.

_____

35. Are test results in agreement?

_____

36. What type of pathology might cause this pattern of audiologic function? Explain how the overall pattern of results would lead you to this conclusion.

_____

_____

_____

_____

## REFLECTION AND REVIEW

1. Why is it important for the audiologist to verify that test results are in agreement?

_____

_____

_____

2. What should the audiologist do if he or she determines that test results are not in agreement?

_____

_____

_____

# ‖‖ 21 ‖‖

## Counseling the Patient

Counseling is the foundation of the interaction with the patient. From this interaction, the clinician learns about the needs and wants of the patient. It is also from this interaction that the patient learns about how his or her hearing loss is impacting communication, what options for treatment are available, and how best to adjust to life with hearing loss.

Your counseling skills will be a large factor in whether a patient has a positive experience with you. We all have had experiences where we felt heard and understood. Likewise, we all have had experiences where we felt "lectured to" and "told what to do." Overall, interacting with a person who genuinely listens and interacts with you is what each of us desires.

In addition to positive affective experiences, the patient also should be informed by your counseling. The needs and wants of the patient should be addressed by your counseling. Information should be presented in such a manner that patients are able to accurately discuss their issues with friends and family members and make appropriate decisions regarding future care.

## LEARNING OUTCOMES

■ Understand the qualities of a good counselor.
■ Be able to present audiologic information in a counseling session.
■ Be able to convey recommendations to a patient.

## REVIEW OF CONCEPTS

### What Makes a Good Counselor?

There are many different skills related to effective counseling. These include the ability to

■ be genuine;
■ understand your own strengths and weaknesses;
■ keep matters confidential;
■ practice focused listening;
■ be nonjudgmental;
■ adapt;
■ see things from new perspectives;
■ communicate;

- apply understanding of gender, generational, and cultural differences; and
- apply audiologic knowledge to benefit the patient.

This chapter focuses on your ability to communicate and to interface your audiologic knowledge and skills with patient needs. Overall, this takes more of an informational approach to counseling. Remember, however, that not all patient counseling is about dissemination of information. It is important to relate to your patient first as a person. The individual's hearing loss is important to the patient only in how it impacts the patient. It is critical that you remember to

- listen to your patient;
- address the patient's questions and needs;
- allow time for the patient to respond;
- allow for silence in the interaction; and
- come to understand the unique characteristics and qualities of your patient, and to address the patient as an individual.

## Using Audiologic Knowledge

The clinician should have a thorough understanding of all tests performed, know how to describe the tests without technical jargon, and know how to explain the results of the testing in meaningful terms. For the patient, meaning stems from issues of communication function, rather than impairment alone. It will not typically be necessary to address every aspect of the testing with patients. In fact, in many cases it would be counterproductive to the patient genuinely understanding the answer to their primary concerns, the meaning of results, prognosis, and next steps. (Consider how much time it took for you to understand how the audiogram and immittance results depict hearing function when you were first exposed.) Nevertheless, you should be able to explain each aspect for those select cases in which a description is important or necessary. Some skills that the audiologist must possess for providing informational counseling include the following:

- Be able to describe the audiogram itself. Typically, the clinician should use words such as

*pitch* versus "frequency," and *loudness* versus "intensity." If the clinician shows the audiogram to the patient, the patient should be oriented to the fact that "low-pitch sounds are on the left side and high-pitch sounds are on the right side of the graph. Very soft sounds are at the top of the graph, and very loud sounds are at the bottom of the graph. The symbols marked on the graph represent the very softest sounds that you can hear."

- Be able to describe location of pathology. When comparing or contrasting bone-conducted and air-conducted signals, or explaining the location of pathology, it is beneficial to have a schematic of the auditory anatomy to show a patient exactly what you mean in your descriptions.
- Be able to provide appropriate and consistent terminology for the patient to describe his or her hearing loss. Be prepared to discuss what these terms mean with your patient.
- Be able to describe to the patient how the hearing loss impacts communication. Descriptions of how different degrees and configurations of hearing loss impact speech understanding are helpful to most patients. A picture of the "speech banana" with a superimposed audiogram, and an audiogram with everyday sounds may be useful to show a patient how his or her hearing loss impacts audibility of sounds. It also may be helpful to discuss with the patient the difference between audibility of sound and clarity of sound. For each of these tasks, the clinician should relate information to the patient's description of communication function and difficulties.
- Be able to relate how word recognition scores may or may not relate to the patient's complaints or concerns about understanding speech in a real-world environment. Be prepared to discuss prognosis for success with hearing instruments or other devices based on word recognition scores and other factors.
- Be able to discuss how medical assessment may be necessary given the type or characteristics of the hearing loss.
- Be able to discuss immittance and otoacoustic emissions results in nontechnical terms. Be able to describe the purpose of the testing and what the results mean. A schematic of the anatomy of the ear may be helpful for this purpose.

■ The clinician should be able to provide an overall impression to the patient from all hearing evaluation results. If results are inconsistent across tests, the audiologist should discuss this and make recommendations for further testing and follow-up.

## Conveying Recommendations

As with basic results, your clinical competence and core knowledge are crucial when conveying recommendations to your patients. Some tips include the following:

■ Be prepared for patients/families that may be in denial or need time to grieve about the hearing loss and recommendations. Overloading a patient or family with information when they are not ready to accept it can lead to a wide range of problems. Do not hesitate to ask patients if they need to stop the interaction and come back to deal with the recommendations after they have had more time to process the information they are hearing. However, do not delay the follow-up visit for too long. Instead, set a reasonable time period such as 1 to 3 days. This recommendation is particularly valuable when working with parents who might be learning about their child's hearing loss for the first time.

■ When working with young children, do not hesitate to inform parents that you are gradually learning more about their child during each visit. Explain that as children grow and change, sometimes a clinician's recommendations may change as well, as more is learned about the child and her or his auditory system.

■ Have written materials/recommended websites for your most common recommendations, for the patient and family to review at their own pace.

■ When recommending amplification, help the patient understand why amplification is recommended, provide a general prognosis for use of amplification, and be prepared to answer basic questions about costs, options, and styles.

■ When recommending a retest, make sure that the patient and/or family member understands why you are making this recommendation. Patients should not leave your office simply saying, "They told me to go for more tests." Instead, he or she should be able to understand the specific reason.

■ Explain how you will convey your recommendations and suggestions to other members of the patient's health care team and how long this process will take (e.g., "I'll send this report to your physician later today.")

■ The concept of "teach back" means that the patient explains to you what you have just told the patient. Use of this technique is highly recommended because it will allow you to know whether the patient did accurately understand what you said, and if not, this will allow you to correct any misunderstandings. For example, you can say, "We went over a lot of information that might be new to you. I want to make sure that I explained it well enough. Can you please tell me in your own words about your hearing loss and what we recommend you do next? For instance, what will you tell your husband/wife when he/she asks you about your results?"

## OBSERVATION

1. Observe an experienced clinician counseling a patient regarding test results after audiologic assessment. What terms did the clinician use to help the patient understand the testing? Would you have described the testing in any different way?

2. Observe the clinician making recommendations with a patient after testing. Were the recommendations clear? Did the patient exhibit an understanding of what to do next? Did the patient appear to "accept" the recommendations? How do you know if the patient understood?

## GUIDED PRACTICE

1. Describe the audiogram to a classmate, friend, or family member.

2. Describe an audiogram with normal audiometric results to a volunteer.

3. Counsel a volunteer with hearing loss.

    a. Describe the audiogram assuming your volunteer has not had a comprehensive audiologic examination before.

    b. Include results from all portions of the test including air- and bone-conduction thresholds, word recognition, and speech reception thresholds.

    c. Describe how you anticipate the results might impact the patient's communication.

    d. Make appropriate recommendations for follow-up testing, hearing instruments, or other considerations.

    e. Give your volunteer an opportunity to ask questions.

    f. Think about how you would change your descriptions if the patient were returning for follow-up testing, or if the volunteer had a long history of hearing aid use.

4. Describe immittance results to a volunteer.

    a. Describe a tympanogram with normal results.

    b. Describe an abnormal tympanogram.

    c. Describe acoustic reflex testing with normal results.

    d. Describe abnormal acoustic reflex test results.

5. After practicing these activities with volunteers, perform these activities with a real patient, under the supervision and guidance of a seasoned clinician.

## REFLECTION AND REVIEW

1. Why is it important to remember to give your patient time to ask questions and reiterate information?

   _____

   _____

   _____

   _____

2. How will your counseling be different for someone who is experiencing a comprehensive audiologic assessment for the first time, versus a patient who is returning to the clinic after many years of assessments?

   _____

   _____

   _____

3. What can you do to be certain that the patient understands the information that you are giving to them?

   _____

   _____

   _____

4. How might your counseling be different for the various patients/families listed below?

   a. The family of an infant with hearing loss

   _____

   _____

   _____

   _____

b. The patient in denial about hearing loss

_____

_____

_____

_____

c. The patient who has accepted the hearing loss and is actively seeking your advice and recommendations

_____

_____

_____

_____

5. How will you incorporate the information gleaned from a referral into your counseling?

_____

_____

_____

_____

6. Why is effective counseling so important?

_____

_____

_____

_____

# ||| 22 |||

## Reporting Results

## INTRODUCTION

Accurate documentation and reporting of results and recommendations is critical. Errors in reporting can be costly to the patient's health and well-being. This chapter focuses on skills in reporting clinical information to patients, families, and other health care providers. Reports such as those used for medical-legal evaluation, which are significantly more detailed, are not addressed in this chapter.

## LEARNING OUTCOMES

- Understand the difference between documenting and reporting.
- Know the fundamental components of reporting results.
- Know how to structure the report that you are writing.
- Be able to create a draft of a report for a hearing evaluation.

## REVIEW OF CONCEPTS

### Documentation Versus Reporting

Documentation of health care information is the means by which information is collected and stored for future reference. Reporting involves the communication of the provider's interpretation of health care information for diagnostic and treatment purposes. Most audiologic reports will contain both interpreted information and documentation. What characterizes truly effective communication is the ability to utilize health care information and test results to make statements regarding function and provide recommendations. Therefore, the focus of the audiologist's report will be the statements regarding function and recommendations. Additional information, in the form of documentation, typically should be included at the end, or as an addendum to the report.

### Why Is Reporting Important?

Reporting is one of the primary ways that you convey information to a referral source or other professionals about a patient's hearing function and recommendations. In many cases, the report you have written will be the only information that another health care provider has about your clinical encounter. The information conveyed in a report often is used by other medical professionals to assist in diagnosis of the patient. Other professionals may use information from the report to determine need for additional supportive services. Therefore, the audiologist's assessment of the patient's hearing function and the recommendations provided by the audiologist are critical in promoting effective patient care. If reporting is poor or sloppy, or does not provide a clear answer to the reader, it can create confusion and impact patient care detrimentally.

## With Whom Are You Communicating?

Communicating with other health care providers will be different than communicating with patients. Patients typically will have less clinical knowledge and will require significantly less technical jargon. With many health care professionals, a certain level of knowledge may be assumed. Depending on the provider, different levels of technical information should be used. A primary care physician or pediatrician will require more explanation and less detail than an otologist.

It would be ideal to write a report with a specific reader in mind, but it is often the case that the report may be read by a number of different consumers. In most current health care settings, medical records are stored electronically. Under current federal guidelines for "meaningful use" of health care data, patients are expected to have access to their own records. In many cases your patient's report may be accessed by them, or by any other relevant physician or provider in a health care setting. Because of this, it is typically best to write the report so that a layperson could understand the information. In addition to providing results and recommendation in clear language, a statement of what results mean for the patient is important. For example, how does a moderate sensorineural hearing loss affect the patient's ability to communicate? For those readers who are more familiar with the specific tests and results, such as an otologist, the attached documentation will provide the detailed results that they need, and they can look to that information directly.

## What to Include?

When reporting information, you should begin with the end in mind. What is it about the clinical encounter that you wish to convey? What brought the patient to you, and how are you working to contribute either a solution or critical information to the care of the patient? The purpose of the report is to tell the story of the patient. An effective interview will be the cornerstone of your clinical reporting. Refer to Chapter 2 for a review of these concepts and methods.

Next, consider the items that are less important. These should receive a different level of treatment in your reporting. For instance, perhaps there is helpful information about the patient that is not absolutely critical to the diagnosis but that lends supporting information to your recommendations. This type of information should be included on a secondary level in your reporting. Details regarding testing parameters are also included at this level.

Finally, consider the details that are unimportant. Although it is tempting to report on every single detail of the clinical encounter, to make sure that you do not "miss anything," too much information does not help the consumer of your information. In many cases, an overabundance of information serves to mask the most important aspects of your report. Obviously, information that does not contribute to improving the reader's understanding should be omitted.

## Elements of the Report

Reports may include the following information:

- Case history: Include items that are relevant to the patient's case and condition.
- Otoscopic inspection: Highlight any abnormalities.

- Immittance results: Highlight abnormalities, and convey how these results complement the other testing you have conducted.
- Otoacoustic emissions: Indicate how these results help to confirm other testing results.
- The audiogram: Describe the
  - type of hearing loss,
  - degree of hearing loss,
  - configuration of hearing loss, and
  - symmetry of hearing loss.
- Speech audiometry: Highlight abnormalities and how these results relate to the hearing loss in question.
- Changes in hearing status (where applicable).
- Reliability of results if there are issues surrounding functional hearing loss.
- Recommendations: Outline the need for further referrals (i.e., medical follow-up, hearing aid evaluation/evaluation for assistive devices, speech and language evaluation).

## GUIDED PRACTICE

Observe a complete evaluation with an experienced audiologist. Then review the reporting completed by the audiologist.

1. Note the structure of the report. Where does it begin? Does it address the situation by "beginning with the end"?

2. How does the report readily identify the information for the reader? Are there different sections that are clearly identified?

3. Are the recommendations clear and based on the evaluation and history data in the report?

4. Perform a complete hearing test evaluation, and write a formal report regarding results.

## REFLECTION AND REVIEW

1. What would the impact be if the patient did not have a clear understanding of her or his hearing loss and recommendations?

_____

_____

_____

2. Why should reports have consistent formats?

_____

_____

_____

3. How do you decide which information is not critical to include in a report?

_____

_____

_____

# ||| 23 |||

## Common Pitfalls in Audiologic Evaluation

### INTRODUCTION

Audiologists can encounter many pitfalls in daily practice. It is important to remember that it is possible for any professional to make a mistake. However, clinical errors can be costly to patients, organizations, and even the audiologist her- or himself. Therefore, it is important to minimize opportunities for errors as much as possible.

### LEARNING OUTCOMES

■ Identify common scenarios in which errors occur during audiologic evaluation.
■ Develop strategies to avoid or remedy errors and challenges that commonly occur.

### REVIEW OF CONCEPTS

The following examples demonstrate some of the challenges that you might encounter in clinical practice.

#### The Patient History

1. Not establishing a rapport with the patient and maintaining eye contact during the interaction. Providers who simply type into a computer while talking with a patient run the risk of not gaining the trust of the patient or family. As a communication professional, you should be modeling appropriate communication behaviors for your patients.
2. Talking with an interpreter versus the patient her- or himself. Always be mindful that the patient is visiting you for the encounter, and

any interpreter is there for best access to communication.

3. Being too scripted during a case history. Occasionally, providers may get lost in following all of the questions on a form versus talking with the patient. Do your best to allow the conversation to flow versus following an overly rehearsed history. In addition, do not ask questions that the patient has already answered simply to follow the order of a form or software program.

4. Making assumptions about a case without verifying the facts with the patient. Remember to consistently check your assumptions and biases.

## Otoscopic Examination

1. Forgetting standard infection control procedure. Although beyond the scope of this manual, you should be conducting all testing with clean hands (and, in some facilities gloves will be required). Your equipment must be clean as well.

2. Forgetting to brace the patient's head appropriately while conducting the otoscopic examination. Your patient could move suddenly and the tip of the otoscope could damage the ear or ear canal causing more bleeding than you might expect. Always brace the head appropriately, particularly with children.

## Audiometry

1. Placing the headphones on the patient and then offering instructions. If you are standing in front of the patient, make sure to instruct him or her with the headphones off of his or her head so that there is every opportunity to hear your instructions clearly.

2. Placing the headphones on the wrong ears. Although this sounds like an easy pitfall to fix by simply "converting" all of the right ear responses to the left side, it can prove complicated, especially when masking. If you make an error and place the headphones incorrectly, it is best to change it right away.

3. Not placing the headphones on the patient at all. Although this sounds nearly impossible, many seasoned providers will tell you that they have accidentally forgotten to place the headphones on a patient once in their careers.

4. Placement of the bone conductor. Always monitor the placement of the bone vibrator on the patient's head. Sometimes the bone conductor will "drift" during testing. Additionally, a patient who wears a wig or other headdress may need to remove it in order for best placement.

5. Intermittent equipment. Rarely, you may deliver a signal and find that the patient does not respond, even at maximum levels. Even though this could be a case of malingering, it could also simply be that there is a short in a cord or a transducer. Confirm that your equipment is working properly before continuing with intense sound levels. Also, use the talkback monitor to listen for the signal in the booth.

6. Routing the signal to the wrong transducer. Check your equipment settings continually during testing, but especially if your results are not what you anticipate.

7. Forgetting to test interoctave frequencies. Remember to test interoctave frequencies whenever you have a 20 dB or greater difference between adjacent octave frequencies on the audiogram.

## Masking

1. Failing to verify the ears and transducers where you are delivering signals. If your testing indicates a conductive hearing loss because of an error in routing signals, you are subjecting your patient to unnecessary medical follow-up.

2. Over- or undermasking. Remember the interaural attenuation values for the transducers you are using, and always recheck your "math" to confirm that you have sufficiently masked without providing too much masking. This is time consuming at first, but it will improve as you gain more experience.

3. Not masking when masking is necessary. Review your audiograms carefully and make

certain that you have verified the need to mask or not mask. Once the patient has left your office, you cannot correct this mistake.

4. Forgetting to mask for speech audiometry. Some new clinicians will find that mastering masking technique for pure tones is challenging enough. They then forget to mask for speech testing altogether.

5. Inadequately instructing the patient for masking. Be certain that your instructions to the patient are clear. Masking can be confusing to both the patient and the new clinician.

## Tympanometry

1. Performing the test with the probe against the canal wall. Newer equipment will likely give you an error message, whereas some older equipment may run the test and provide a flat tympanogram. The answer in this situation is to always verify the equivalent ear canal volume. If your reading is "0.0 cm$^3$," you know that you are likely against the canal wall.

2. Failing to instruct the patient adequately. Patients who have never experienced tympanometry may expect there to be pain involved. It is important to reassure the patient that the test is typically painless.

3. Not setting or marking the test ear. Always confirm which ear you are testing, and make sure that your equipment is set appropriately to indicate the correct ear.

## Acoustic Reflexes/ Acoustic Reflex Decay

1. Inappropriately routing the signals. Always make sure that your equipment is set up as you have planned. Confirm which ear is the test ear and that the equipment is routing signals exactly as you have planned.

2. Failure to monitor the intensity of the signals delivered. Be cautious when delivering the signals to the patient's ears. The impedance equipment can produce intense signals that could potentially damage the patient's hearing.

3. Failing to instruct the patient appropriately. It is important to remind the patient that although he or she may be hearing some "loud sounds," the patient does not need to do anything but remain quiet and patient during the testing.

## Otoacoustic Emissions

1. Testing with the probe plugged. Be cautious that even a slight amount of cerumen or debris in the ear canal can cause the OAE probe to become plugged, interfering with the ability to present a stimulus or to record a response.

2. Failure to monitor the intensity of the signals delivered. Equipment problems or a poorly fit probe tip can result in an inappropriate intensity of signal delivered to the ear canal. Monitoring the stimulus intensity can also alert the clinician when a probe has fallen out of the ear canal.

## Counseling

1. Rushing through counseling. It is important that your patient understands your findings and recommendations. Take the extra moment to confirm the patient's knowledge and understanding before he or she leaves the office.

2. Forgetting critical recommendations. Nearly every audiologist has forgotten to make a recommendation clear to a patient or family member. It is your responsibility to relay all pertinent information to your patient. If you have forgotten something, it is your professional role to contact the patient personally.

3. Poorly documenting your counseling encounter. Your documentation protects the patient and yourself. Make certain that all of your recommendations are accurately recorded in the patient's record.

4. Using jargon or complex terminology. Always remember that you are the professional, and your patient does not have a deep understanding of the auditory system. It is your responsibility to be clear, direct, and appropriate in your communication with a patient. Some patients will be able to understand more

jargon (perhaps those who work in the medical field) versus the average patient.

5. Focusing all of your energy on family members and not the patient. Be mindful of who is visiting you. Occasionally, new providers may forget that elderly patients are very capable of interacting with professionals, and the new provider may spend her or his efforts on the adult child or caregiver who is present with the patient. Think of your patient first, and involve family members or caregivers where appropriate.

6. Offering too much information all at once. Be mindful of how much information a patient is ready to comprehend. Written materials and follow-up visits may be necessary over time.

### Final Thoughts

Although it may appear that there are many opportunities for mistakes in a patient encounter, you can mitigate these errors with the use of appropriate written protocols and checklists. Spending the time to determine each step of an encounter can be a fruitful exercise.

## OBSERVATION

1. Observe the language that an audiologist uses when talking with a patient. What terms does he or she change in order to make them "patient friendly"?

2. Ask the audiologist you are observing if he or she has any written protocols he or she is willing to share with you.

3. Carefully observe how and when the audiologist documents the different elements of the encounter. At what points is the documentation occurring?

## REFLECTION AND REVIEW

1. How could having the headphones on the wrong ears be a costly mistake?

_____

_____

_____

2. Describe different ways you could contact a patient if you believed that there was an element of your interaction with him or her that needed more input or clarification. What ways are best, and why?

_____

_____

_____

_____

_____

3. Imagine you have placed the headphones on the wrong ears of your patient. You have made the discovery early in testing. What will you say to your patient as you correct the problem? (*Hint*: How can you not lose the confidence and trust of your patient?)

_____

_____

_____

# References and Bibliography

American National Standards Institute. (2004). *Specifications for audiometers (S3.6-2004)*. New York, NY: Acoustical Society of America.

Cranford, J. L. (2007). *Basics of audiology: From vibration to sound*. San Diego, CA: Plural.

Dhar, S., & Hall, J. W., III. (2012). *Otoacoustic emissions: Principles, procedures, and protocols*. San Diego, CA: Plural.

Hall, J. W., III, & Swanepoel, D. (2010). *Objective assessment of hearing*. San Diego, CA: Plural.

Huff, S. J., & Nerbonne, M. A. (1982). Comparison of the American Speech-Language-Hearing Association and revised Tillman-Olsen methods for speech threshold measurement. *Ear and Hearing, 3*, 335–339.

Hunter, L. L., & Shahnaz, N. (2014). *Acoustic immittance measures: Basic and advanced practice*. San Diego, CA: Plural.

Katz, J., & Lezynski, J. (2002). Clinical masking. In J. Katz (Ed.), *Handbook of clinical audiology*. (pp. 124–141). Philadelphia, PA: Lippincott Williams & Wilkins.

Killion, M. C., Wilber, L. A., & Gudmundsen, G. I. (1985). Insert earphones for more interaural attenuation. *Hearing Instruments, 36*, 34–36.

Lawson, G., & Peterson, M. (2011). *Speech audiometry*. San Diego, CA: Plural.

Margolis, R. H., & Hunter, L. L. (2000). Acoustic immittance measurements. In R. Roeser, M. Valente, & H. Hosford-Dunn (Eds.), *Audiology: Diagnosis* (pp. 381–424). New York, NY: Thieme Medical.

Martin, F. (2009). Nonorganic hearing loss. In J. Katz, L. Medwetsky, R. Burkard, & L. Hood (Eds.), *Handbook of clinical audiology* (6th ed., pp. 699–711). Baltimore, MD: Lippincott Williams & Wilkins.

Pasha, R. (2006). *Otolaryngology head and neck surgery: Clinical reference guide* (2nd ed.). San Diego, CA: Plural.

Ramachandran, V., & Stach, B. A. (2013). *Professional communication in audiology*. San Diego, CA: Plural.

Stach, B. A. (2008). Reporting audiometric results. *Hearing Journal, 61*(9), 10–16.

Stach, B. A. (2010). *Clinical audiology: An introduction* (2nd ed.). Clifton Park, NY: Delmar, Cengage Learning.

Studebaker, G. A. (1979). Clinical masking. In W. F. Rintelmann (Ed.), *Hearing assessment*. Baltimore, MD: University Park Press.

Touma, J., & Touma, B. (2006). *Atlas of otoscopy*. San Diego, CA: Plural.

Valente, M. (2009). *Pure-tone audiometry and masking*. San Diego, CA: Plural.

Wiley, T. L., & Fowler, C. G. (1997). *Acoustic immittance measures in clinical audiology: A primer*. San Diego, CA: Singular.

Yacullo, W. S. (1996). *Clinical masking procedures*. Boston, MA: Allyn & Bacon.

# Index

**Note:** Page numbers in **bold** reference non-text material.